FIVE-STAR

SOUTH CAROLINA UPSTATE

Five-Star Trails: South Carolina Upstate
Spectacular Hikes Near Greenville, Spartanburg, Oconee, and Pickens Counties

Published by Menasha Ridge Press
Distributed by Publishers Group West
Printed in China
First edition, 2013; second edition, 2023

Editors: Holly Cross and Andrew Mollenkof
Cover design: Scott McGrew
Text design: Annie Long
Cover and interior photos: Sherry Jackson
Cartography and elevation profiles: Sherry Jackson and Steve Jones
Indexer: Rich Carlson

Library of Congress Cataloging-in-Publication Data
  Names: Jackson, Sherry (Information technology professional), author.
  Title: Five star trails South Carolina upstate : spectacular hikes near Greenville, Spartanburg, Oconee,
    and Pickens Counties / Sherry Jackson.
  Other titles: South Carolina upstate | 5 star trails South Carolina upstate
  Description: 2nd Edition. | Birmingham, AL : Menasha Ridge Press, [2023] | Series: Five-star trails
    "1st edition 2013"—T.p. verso.
  Identifiers: LCCN 2022049807 (print) | LCCN 2022049808 (ebook) | ISBN 9781634043465 (Paperback)
    ISBN 9781634043472 (eBook)
  Subjects: LCSH: Hiking—South Carolina—Guidebooks. | Trails—South Carolina—Guidebooks.
    South Carolina—Guidebooks.
  Classification: LCC GV199.42.S58 J33 2023 (print) | LCC GV199.42.S58 (ebook)
    DDC 796.5109757—dc23/eng/20230103
  LC record available at https://lccn.loc.gov/2022049807
  LC ebook record available at https://lccn.loc.gov/2022049808

 MENASHA RIDGE PRESS
An imprint of AdventureKEEN
2204 First Ave. S., Ste. 102
Birmingham, AL 35233
800-678-7006, fax 877-374-9016

Visit menasharidge.com for a complete listing of our books and for ordering information. Contact us at our website, at facebook.com/menasharidge, or at twitter.com/menasharidge with questions or comments. To find out more about who we are and what we're doing, visit blog.menasharidge.com.

SAFETY NOTICE Though the author and publisher have made every effort to ensure that the information in this book is accurate at press time, they are not responsible for any loss, damage, injury, or inconvenience that may occur while using this book—you are responsible for your own safety and health on the trail. The fact that a hike is described in this book does not mean that it will be safe for you. Always check local conditions (which can change from day to day), know your own limitations, and consult a map.

For information about trail and other closures, check the "Contact" listings in the hike profiles.

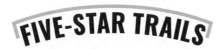

FIVE-STAR TRAILS

SOUTH CAROLINA UPSTATE

SPECTACULAR HIKES
Near Greenville, Spartanburg, Oconee, and Pickens Counties

SHERRY JACKSON

MENASHA RIDGE PRESS

South Carolina Upstate Overview Map

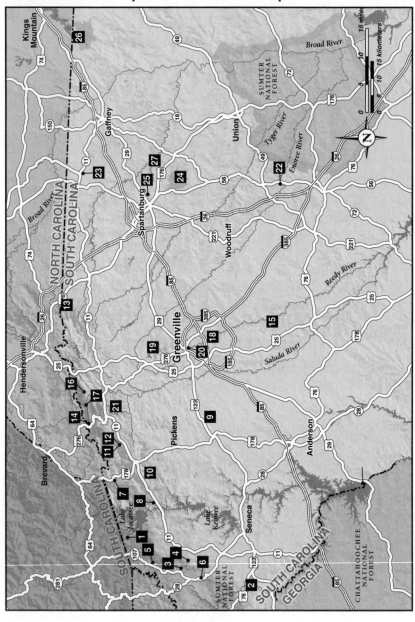

Contents

Dedication

This book is for everyone who enjoys hiking the gorgeous and varied landscape in the Upstate of South Carolina.

 # Acknowledgments

SPECIAL THANKS GO TO MY HUSBAND, PHIL, who trekked every single mile with me, again; my son, Justin; and my family and friends who kept encouraging me. A special shout-out to the park rangers who helped me along the way and the volunteers and outdoor enthusiasts who keep our beautiful trails in the Upstate maintained so everyone can enjoy them.

—Sherry Jackson

Preface

WHEN MY PUBLISHER CONTACTED ME TO DO AN UPDATE TO THIS HIKING GUIDE, I had just returned to South Carolina after a three-year stint in Arizona. I had desperately missed the people, mountains, trails, and lakes of the Upstate. Coming back was a true homecoming. This is where I'm meant to be.

The trail system in the Upstate is quite extensive, and hikes range from day hikes, covered in the following pages, to multiday hikes along the Foothills and Appalachian Trails. Our trails are diverse, ranging from easy paths just minutes away from metropolitan areas to strenuous trails where you feel more like you are climbing mountains. And the views—well, they're downright incredible. We have some of the best mountains and parks in the South, and our many breathtaking waterfalls lure hikers to the trails.

In this second edition, I've included some new trails I've discovered and discarded some that weren't quite up to par. As before, I tried to include a good variety of easy, moderate, and strenuous hikes in all areas of the Upstate's six counties. All of the trips I've chosen can be done by any able-bodied person. I love to hike, but I've never been athletic—so if I can do it, *you* can do it. Get outside and hit the trails!

—S. J.

Recommended Hikes

Best for Dogs

13 Blue Wall Passage of the Palmetto Trail and Waterfall Loop (p. 78)

25 Edwin M. Griffin Nature Preserve (p. 130)

27 Pacolet River Heritage Trust Preserve: Lawson's Fork Trail (p. 140)

Best for Fall Color

2 Chau Ram County Park (p. 23)

10 Nine Times Preserve (p. 62)

19 Paris Mountain State Park: Brissy Ridge Trail (p. 102)

Best for History

22 Battle of Musgrove Mill State Historic Site: British Camp and Battlefield Trails (p. 118)

23 Cowpens Battlefield Trail (p. 122)

26 Kings Mountain (p. 135)

Best for Kids

4 Oconee Station: Interpretive Nature Trail and Station Cove Trail (p. 31)

9 Nalley Brown Nature Park: Nalley Trail (p. 58)

20 Swamp Rabbit Trail: Cleveland Park to Linky Stone Park (p. 107)

24 Croft State Park Nature Trail (p. 126)

Best for Nature

3 Oconee State Park: Old Waterwheel Trail (p. 27)

7 Eastatoe Creek Heritage Preserve Trail (p. 48)

11 Table Rock State Park: Carrick Creek Trail (p. 66)

16 Jones Gap State Park: Falls Trail (p. 90)

18 Lake Conestee Nature Preserve (p. 98)

Best for Scenery

8 Keowee-Toxaway State Park: Raven Rock Trail (p. 52)

12 Table Rock State Park: Table Rock Trail (p. 71)

14 Caesars Head State Park: Raven Cliff Falls (p. 82)

Best for Seclusion

1 Bad Creek: Lower Whitewater Falls Trail (p. 18)

7 Eastatoe Creek Heritage Preserve Trail (p. 48)

Best for Waterfalls

1 Bad Creek: Lower Whitewater Falls Trail (p. 18)

6 Yellow Branch Falls (p. 40)

11 Table Rock State Park: Carrick Creek Trail (p. 66)

15 Cedar Falls Park Trail (p. 86)

17 Jones Gap State Park: Rainbow Falls Trail (p. 94)

21 Wildcat Branch Falls Trail (p. 112)

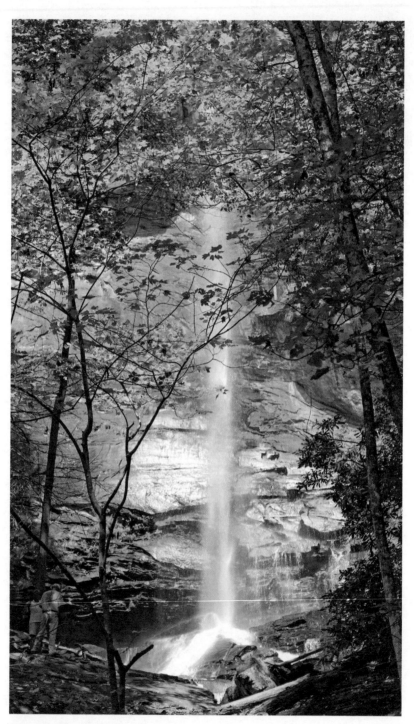

RAINBOW FALLS AT JONES GAP STATE PARK *(See Hike 17, page 94.)*

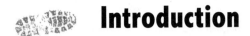 # Introduction

About This Book

Five Star Trails: South Carolina Upstate features 27 spectacular hikes near Greenville, Spartanburg, Oconee, and Pickens Counties. Thank you for picking up the second edition of this book, which features several new hikes, along with some updates to popular trails that have changed course.

While the criteria vary regarding which counties are officially part of the Upstate, I've focused on the six main counties, grouping them into four sections as you would travel: from Anderson and Oconee Counties in the state's western terrain northward to Pickens County, then arcing eastward to Greenville and, finally, swooping northeastward to Spartanburg and Cherokee Counties. Together, these locations create a broad semicircle from the Georgia border up and around just south of the North Carolina line.

★ **Anderson County** includes the city of Anderson. **Oconee County** sits at the foothills of the Blue Ridge Mountains. Often referred to as the Mountain Lakes region, the area is home to world-class lakes, rivers, parks, and waterfalls.

★ **Pickens County,** the gateway to the mountainous region of the Upstate, contains perhaps some of the greatest scenery and hiking adventures, with Table Rock State Park, Lake Keowee, and Lake Jocassee.

★ **Greenville County** ranks largest in the Upstate and includes the cities of Greenville, Mauldin, Simpsonville, and Travelers Rest. A major portion of Upstate residents can easily reach trails in this area for an after-work or quick weekend jaunt.

★ **Spartanburg County** is the second largest in the Upstate in terms of population. "Born from the revolution," this county is home to Musgrove Mill, a significant Revolutionary War site. Its companion in this book, **Cherokee County,** encompasses anything north of Spartanburg and includes Cowpens and Kings Mountain, both significant historical sites.

How to Use This Guidebook

Overview Map, Regional Maps, and Map Legend

The overview map on page iv depicts the location of the primary trailhead for all of the hikes described in this book. The numbers shown on the overview map pair with the table of contents on the facing page. Each hike's number is also listed in the corresponding regional chapter's table of contents and overview map, as well as on the opening page of each hike profile. The four regional overview maps provide more detail than the main overview map, bringing you closer to the hikes in their respective chapters. A legend explaining the map symbols used throughout the book appears below.

Trail Maps

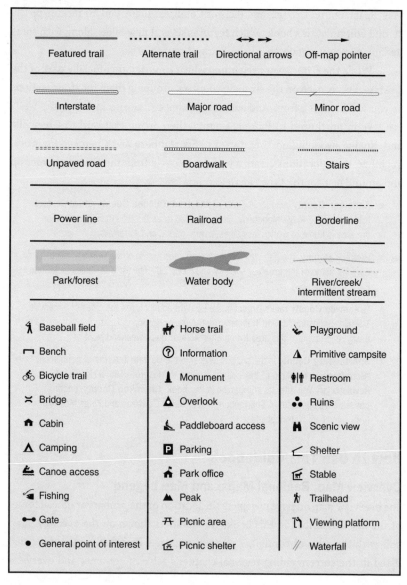

Featured trail	Alternate trail	Directional arrows	Off-map pointer

Interstate	Major road	Minor road

Unpaved road	Boardwalk	Stairs

Power line	Railroad	Borderline

Park/forest	Water body	River/creek/intermittent stream

Baseball field	Horse trail	Playground
Bench	Information	Primitive campsite
Bicycle trail	Monument	Restroom
Bridge	Overlook	Ruins
Cabin	Paddleboard access	Scenic view
Camping	Parking	Shelter
Canoe access	Park office	Stable
Fishing	Peak	Trailhead
Gate	Picnic area	Viewing platform
General point of interest	Picnic shelter	Waterfall

In addition to the overview and regional maps, a detailed map of each hike's route appears with its profile. On this map, symbols indicate the trailhead, the complete route, significant features, facilities, and topographic landmarks such as creeks, overlooks, and peaks.

To produce the highly accurate maps in this book, I used a handheld GPS unit to gather data while hiking each route, then sent that data to the publisher's cartographers. However, your GPS is not a substitute for sound, sensible navigation that considers the conditions you observe while hiking.

Further, despite the high quality of the maps in this guidebook, the publisher and I strongly recommend you always carry an additional map, such as the ones noted in each profile opener's "Maps" listing.

Elevation Profile

This diagram represents the rises and falls of the trail as viewed from the side, over the complete distance (in miles) of that trail. On the diagram's vertical axis, or height scale, the number of feet indicated between each tick mark lets you visualize the climb. To avoid making flat hikes look steep and steep hikes appear flat, varying height scales provide an accurate image of each hike's climbing challenge. For example, one hike's scale might rise from 1,145 feet to 3,134 feet, as on the Table Rock Trail (see Hike 12, page 71), while the Musgrove Mill trails (Hike 22, page 118) start at 396 and 433 feet and go only to 524 and 529 feet. Not all hikes include an elevation profile, especially relatively flat greenways and lake loops.

The Hike Profile

Each profile opens with the hike's star ratings, trailhead GPS coordinates, and other key information—from the trail's distance and configuration to contacts for local information. Each profile also includes a map (see "Trail Maps," above). The main text for each profile includes four sections: Overview, Route Details, Nearby Attractions, and Directions (for driving to the trailhead area). See page 6 for more information.

Star Ratings

Following is the explanation for the rating system of one to five stars in each of the five categories for each hike.

FOR SCENERY:

★★★★★	Unique, picturesque panoramas
★★★★	Diverse vistas
★★★	Pleasant views
★★	Unchanging landscape
★	Not selected for scenery

FOR TRAIL CONDITION:

★★★★★	Consistently well maintained
★★★★	Stable, with no surprises
★★★	Average terrain to negotiate
★★	Inconsistent, with good and poor areas
★	Rocky, overgrown, or often muddy

FOR CHILDREN:

★★★★★	Babes in strollers are welcome
★★★★	Fun for any kid past the toddler stage
★★★	Good for young hikers with proven stamina
★★	Not enjoyable for children
★	Not advisable for children

FOR DIFFICULTY:

★★★★★	Grueling
★★★★	Strenuous
★★★	Moderate—won't beat you up, but you'll know you've been hiking
★★	Easy, with patches of moderate
★	Good for a relaxing stroll

FOR SOLITUDE:

★★★★★	Positively tranquil
★★★★	Spurts of isolation
★★★	Moderately secluded
★★	Crowded on weekends and holidays
★	Steady stream of individuals and/or groups

TRAILHEAD GPS COORDINATES

As noted in "Trail Maps," on the previous page, I used a handheld GPS unit to obtain geographic data and sent the information to the publisher's cartographers. In the opener for each hike profile, the coordinates—the intersection of latitude (north) and longitude (west)—will orient you from the trailhead. In some cases, you can drive within viewing distance of a trailhead. Other hiking routes require a short walk to the trailhead from a parking area.

This guidebook uses the degree–decimal minute format for presenting the GPS coordinates. The latitude and longitude grid system is likely quite familiar to you, but here is a refresher, pertinent to visualizing the GPS coordinates: Imaginary lines of latitude—called *parallels* and approximately 69 miles apart from each other—run horizontally around the globe. Each parallel is indicated by degrees from the equator (established to be 0°): up to 90°N at the North Pole and down to 90°S at the South Pole.

Imaginary lines of longitude—called *meridians*—run perpendicular to latitude lines. Longitude lines are likewise indicated by degrees: starting from 0° at the Prime Meridian in Greenwich, England, they continue to the east and west until they meet 180° later at the International Date Line in the Pacific Ocean. At the equator, longitude lines are also approximately 69 miles apart, but that distance narrows as the meridians converge toward the North and South Poles.

To convert GPS coordinates given in degrees, minutes, and seconds to the format shown above in degrees–decimal minutes, divide the seconds by 60. For more on GPS technology, visit usgs.gov.

DISTANCE & CONFIGURATION

Distance indicates the length of the hike from start to finish, either round-trip or one-way depending on the trail configuration. If the hike description includes options to shorten or extend the hike, those distances will also be factored here. Configuration defines the type of route—for example, an out-and-back (which takes you in and out the same way), a figure eight, a loop, or a balloon.

HIKING TIME

I'm not the fastest hiker, and that was especially true while I was updating this book. I had to stop and take notes—a lot. Thus, the average of 1.3 miles per hour for the hikes in this guidebook might be slower than what you're used to. That pace allows time for taking photos, for dawdling and admiring views, and for alternating stretches of hills and descents. When deciding whether to follow a particular trail in this guidebook, consider the weather, your own pace, your general physical condition, and your energy level that day. Remember that daylight hours during late fall through early spring are limited, so plan accordingly to make sure you don't end up on the trail after dark.

HIGHLIGHTS

Waterfalls, historic sites, and other features that draw hikers to the trail are emphasized here.

ELEVATION

Here you will see the elevation (in feet) at the trailhead and another figure for the peak height on that route. For routes that involve significant ascents and descents, the hike profile also includes an elevation diagram (see page 3).

ACCESS

Fees or permits required to hike the trail are detailed here—and noted if there are none. Trail access hours are also shown here.

MAPS

Resources for maps, in addition to those in this guidebook, are listed here. (As previously noted, the publisher and author recommend that you carry more than one map—and that you consult those maps before heading out on the trail to resolve any confusion or discrepancy.)

FACILITIES

Restrooms, phones, water, picnic tables, and other basics at or near the trailhead are mentioned here.

WHEELCHAIR ACCESS

Notes paved sections or other areas where one can safely use a wheelchair.

COMMENTS

Here you'll find assorted nuggets of information, such as whether dogs are allowed on the trails.

CONTACTS

Listed here are phone numbers and website addresses for checking trail conditions and gleaning other day-to-day information.

Overview, Route Details, Nearby Attractions, and Directions

These four elements provide the main text about the hike. **Overview** gives you a quick summary of what to expect on that trail; the **Route Details** guide you on the hike, start to finish; **Nearby Attractions** suggests appealing area sites, such as restaurants, museums, and other trails; **Directions** will get you to the trailhead from a well-known road or highway.

Weather

The Upstate of South Carolina has four distinctive seasons. It can be cold in the winter and hot in the summer. You can enjoy hiking trails any time of the year, but a good rule of thumb is to hit the mountains and waterfalls in the warmer months and the urban trails during the cooler ones. Also keep in mind that temperatures can vary significantly: if it's 50°F in Greenville, it could be freezing in Oconee or Pickens County, so always check the weather before you head out.

To give you an idea of what weather to expect, the chart below details the monthly averages for South Carolina's Upstate region.

MONTHLY WEATHER AVERAGES FOR SC UPSTATE

MONTH	HI TEMP	LO TEMP	RAIN OR SNOW
January	50.2°F	31.4°F	4.41"
February	54.8°F	33.9°F	4.24"
March	62.7°F	40.5°F	5.31"
April	71.0°F	47.0°F	3.54"
May	78.2°F	56.2°F	4.59"
June	85.1°F	64.3°F	3.92"
July	88.8°F	68.7°F	4.65"
August	87.1°F	67.9°F	4.08"
September	81.1°F	61.7°F	3.97"
October	71.4°F	49.7°F	3.88"
November	61.3°F	41.0°F	3.79"
December	52.7°F	34.3°F	3.86"

Source: usclimatedata.com

Water

How much is enough? One simple physiological fact should convince you to err on the side of excess when deciding how much water to pack: you can sweat nearly 2 quarts of fluid each hour you walk in the heat, more if you hike uphill in direct sunlight and during the hottest time of the day. A good rule of thumb is to hydrate prior to your hike, carry (and drink) 16 ounces of water for every mile you plan to hike, and hydrate again after the hike. For most people, the pleasures of hiking make carrying water a relatively minor price to pay to remain safe and healthy. So pack more water than you anticipate needing, even for short hikes.

If you are tempted to drink "found" water, do so with extreme caution. Many ponds and lakes you'll encounter are fairly stagnant, and the water tastes terrible. Drinking such water presents inherent risks for thirsty trekkers. Giardia parasites contaminate many water sources and cause the dreaded intestinal ailment giardiasis, which can last for weeks after ingestion. For information, visit the Centers for Disease Control website: cdc.gov/parasites/giardia.

In any case, effective treatment is essential before you drink from any water source found along the trail. Boiling water for 2–3 minutes is always a safe measure for camping, but day hikers can consider iodine tablets, approved chemical mixes, filtration units rated for giardia, and UV filtration. Some of these methods (for example, filtration with an added carbon filter) remove bad tastes typical in stagnant water, while others add their own taste. Carry a means of purification to help in a pinch and if you realize you have underestimated your consumption needs.

Clothing

Weather, unexpected trail conditions, fatigue, extended hiking duration, and wrong turns can individually or collectively turn a great outing into a very uncomfortable one at best—and a life-threatening one at worst. Thus, proper attire plays a key role in staying comfortable and, sometimes, in staying alive. Here are some helpful guidelines:

★ *Choose silk, wool, or synthetics for maximum comfort in all of your hiking attire*— from hats to socks and in between. Cotton is fine if the weather remains dry and stable, but you won't be happy if it gets wet.

★ *Always wear a hat,* or at least tuck one into your day pack or hitch it to your belt. Hats offer all-weather sun and wind protection as well as warmth if it turns cold.

★ *Be ready to layer up or down as the day progresses and the mercury rises or falls.* Today's outdoor wear makes layering easy, with such designs as jackets that convert to vests and zip-off or button-up pant legs.

★ *Wear hiking boots/shoes or sturdy hiking sandals with toe protection.* Flip-flopping on a paved path in an urban botanical garden is one thing, but never hike a trail in open sandals or casual sneakers. Your bones and arches need support, and your skin needs protection.

★ *Pair that footwear with good socks!* If you prefer not to sheathe your feet when wearing hiking sandals, tuck the socks into your day pack; you may need them if the weather plummets or if you hit rocky turf and pebbles begin to irritate your feet. And, in an emergency, if you have lost your gloves, you can use the socks as mittens.

★ *Don't leave rainwear behind,* even if the day dawns clear and sunny. Tuck into your day pack, or tie around your waist, a jacket that is breathable and either water-resistant or waterproof. Investigate different choices at your local outdoor retailer. If you are a frequent hiker, ideally you'll have more than one rainwear weight, material, and style in your closet to protect you in all seasons in your regional climate and hiking microclimates.

Essential Gear

Today you can buy outdoor vests that have up to 20 pockets shaped and sized to carry everything from toothpicks to binoculars. Or, if you don't aspire to feel like a burro, you can neatly stow all these items in your day pack or backpack. The following list showcases never-hike-without-them items—in alphabetical order, as all are important:

★ *Extra clothes:* Raingear, a change of socks and shirt, and depending on the season, a warm hat and gloves

★ *Extra food:* Trail mix, granola bars, or other high-energy foods

★ *Flashlight or headlamp* with an extra bulb and batteries

★ *Insect repellent:* For some areas and seasons, this is extremely vital.

★ *Maps and a high-quality compass:* Even if you know the terrain from previous hikes, don't leave home without these tools. And, as previously noted, bring maps in addition to those in this guidebook, and consult your maps prior to the hike. If you're GPS-savvy, bring that device, too—along with extra batteries—but don't rely on it as your sole navigational tool, as batteries can die. Be sure to compare the guidance of your GPS with that of your maps and compass.

★ *A pocketknife and/or multitool*

★ *Sun protection:* Sunglasses with UV tinting, a hat with a wide brim, and sunscreen (be sure to check the expiration date on the tube or bottle)

★ *Today's handheld devices* have not only a phone that may help you contact help, but also built-in GPS that can help with orientation. However, do not call for help unless you are truly in need, and remember that smartphone batteries can die, though a cell battery pack helps. Additionally, you can use your smartphone to download park maps for reference. However, download maps at home rather than taking chances with reception in the hinterlands. And be sure your device is fully charged before your hike, so you'll have access to your maps for the duration of your hike.

★ *Water:* Again, bring more than you think you'll drink. Depending on your destination, you may want to bring a water bottle and iodine or a filter for purifying water in the wilderness in case you run out.

★ *Whistle:* This little gadget could be your best friend in an emergency.

★ *Windproof matches and/or a lighter,* as well as a fire starter, for real emergencies. Please don't start a forest fire.

First Aid Kit

Combined with the items above, those below may appear overwhelming for a day hike. But any paramedic will tell you that the items listed here (again, in alphabetical order, because all are important) are just the basics. The reality of hiking is that you can be out for a week of backpacking and acquire only a mosquito bite—or you can hike for an hour, slip, and suffer a bleeding abrasion or broken bone. Fortunately, these items will collapse into a very small space, and convenient prepackaged kits are widely available.

Consider your intended terrain and the number of hikers in your party before you exclude any item listed below. A botanical garden stroll may not inspire you to carry a complete kit, but anything beyond that warrants precaution. When hiking alone, you should always be prepared for a medical need. And if you are a twosome or a group, one or more people in your party should be equipped with first aid supplies.

★ *Adhesive bandages (such as Band-Aids)*

★ *Antibiotic ointment (such as Neosporin)*

★ *Athletic tape*

★ *Blister kit (such as Moleskin or Spenco 2nd Skin)*

★ *Butterfly-closure bandages*

★ *Diphenhydramine (Benadryl or the generic equivalent),* in case of mild allergic reactions

★ *Elastic bandages (such as Ace) or joint wraps (such as Spenco)*

★ *Epinephrine in a prefilled syringe (EpiPen),* usually by prescription only, for people known to have severe allergic reactions to hiking mishaps such as bee stings

★ *Gauze (one roll and a half dozen 4-by-4-inch pads)*

★ *Hydrogen peroxide or iodine*

★ *Ibuprofen or acetaminophen*

General Safety

★ *Always let someone know where you will be hiking and how long you expect to be gone.* It's a good idea to give that person a copy of your route, particularly if you are headed into any isolated area. Let that person know when you return.

★ *Always sign in and out of any trail registers provided.* Don't hesitate to comment on the trail condition if space is provided; that's your opportunity to alert others to any problems you encounter.

★ *Do not count on a smartphone for your safety.* Reception may be spotty or nonexistent on the trail, even on an urban walk—especially if it's embraced by towering trees or buildings.

★ *Always carry food and water, even for a short hike.* And bring more water than you think you will need. (We can't emphasize this enough!)

★ *Stay on designated trails.* Even on the most clearly marked trails, there is usually a point where you must stop and consider in which direction to head. If you become disoriented, don't panic. As soon as you think you may be off track, stop, assess your current direction, and then retrace your steps to the point where you went astray. Using a map, a compass, a GPS, and this book, and keeping in mind what you have passed thus far, reorient yourself and trust your judgment on which way to continue. Also, see if your smartphone or handheld device has map capability and use it for orientation. If you become unsure of how to continue, return to your vehicle the way you came in. Should you become completely lost and have no idea how to return to the trailhead, remaining in place along the trail and waiting for help is most often the best option for adults and always the best option for children.

★ *Always carry a whistle,* another precaution that we can't overemphasize. It may be a lifesaver if you get lost or hurt.

★ *Be especially careful when crossing streams.* Whether you are fording the stream or crossing on a log, make every step count. If you have any doubt about maintaining your balance on a log, ford the stream instead: use a trekking pole or stout stick for balance and face upstream as you cross. If a stream seems too deep to ford, turn back. Whatever is on the other side is not worth risking your life for.

★ *Be careful at overlooks.* While these areas may provide spectacular views, they are potentially hazardous. Stay back from the edge of outcrops and be absolutely sure of your footing; a misstep can mean a nasty and possibly fatal fall.

★ *Standing dead trees and storm-damaged living trees pose a significant hazard to hikers.* These trees may have loose or broken limbs that could fall at any time. While walking beneath trees, and when choosing a spot to rest or enjoy your snack, **look up!**

★ *Know the symptoms of subnormal body temperature (hypothermia).* Shivering and forgetfulness are the two most common indicators of this stealthy killer. Hypothermia can occur at any elevation, even in the summer, especially when the hiker is wearing lightweight cotton clothing. If symptoms present themselves, get to shelter, hot liquids, and dry clothes as soon as possible.

★ *Know the symptoms of heat exhaustion (hyperthermia).* Lightheadedness and loss of energy are the first two indicators. If you feel these symptoms, find some shade, drink your water, remove as many layers of clothing as practical, and stay put until you cool down. Marching through heat exhaustion leads to heatstroke—which can be fatal. If you should be sweating and you're not, that's the signature warning sign.

Your hike is over at that point—heatstroke is a life-threatening condition that can cause seizures, convulsions, and eventually death. If you or a companion reaches that point, do whatever you can to cool down and find help.

★ *Ask questions.* Public-land employees are there to help. It's a lot easier to ask advice beforehand, and it will help you avoid a mishap away from civilization when it's too late to amend an error.

★ *Most important of all, take along your brain.* A cool, calculating mind is the single-most important asset on the trail. Think before you act. Watch your step. Plan ahead. Avoiding accidents before they happen is the best way to ensure a rewarding and relaxing hike.

Watchwords for Flora and Fauna

Hikers should remain aware of the following concerns regarding plant life and wildlife, described in alphabetical order.

BLACK BEARS Though attacks by black bears are uncommon, the sight or approach of a bear can give anyone a start. If you encounter a bear while hiking, remain calm and avoid running in any direction. Make loud noises to scare off the bear, and back away slowly. In primitive and remote areas, assume bears are present; in more developed sites, check on the current bear situation prior to hiking. Most encounters are food related, as bears have an exceptional sense of smell and not particularly discriminating tastes. While this is of greater concern to backpackers and campers, on a day hike, you may plan a lunchtime picnic or munch an energy bar or other snack from time to time so remain aware and alert.

MOSQUITOES Ward off these pests with insect repellent and/or repellent-impregnated clothing. In some areas, mosquitoes are known to carry the West Nile virus, so all caution should be taken to avoid their bites.

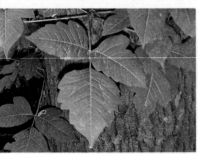

POISON IVY *Tom Watson*

POISON IVY, OAK, AND SUMAC Recognizing and avoiding poison ivy, oak, and sumac is the most effective way to prevent the painful, itchy rashes associated with these plants. Poison ivy occurs as a vine or ground cover, three leaflets to a leaf; poison oak occurs as either a vine or shrub, also with three leaflets; and poison sumac flourishes in swampland, each leaf having 7–13 leaflets. Urushiol, the oil in the sap of these plants, is responsible for the rash. Within 14 hours of exposure, raised lines and/or blisters will appear on the affected area, accompanied by a terrible itch. Refrain from scratching because bacteria under your fingernails can cause an infection. Wash and dry the affected area thoroughly, applying a calamine lotion to help dry out the rash. If itching or blistering is severe, seek medical attention. If you do encounter one of these plants, remember that oil-contaminated clothes, hiking gear, and pets can easily cause an irritating rash on you or someone else, so wash not only any exposed parts of your body but also any exposed clothes, gear, and pets.

SNAKES Rattlesnakes, cottonmouths, copperheads, and corals are among the most common venomous snakes in the United States, and hibernation season is typically October–April. Rattlesnakes like to bask in the sun and won't bite unless threatened. In the Upstate, copperheads, rattlesnakes, and cottonmouths are all indigenous, and while they're not frequently seen on area trails, you still need to keep an eye out for them.

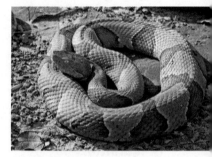

COPPERHEAD
Creeping Things/Shutterstock

However, the snakes you will most likely see while hiking will be non-venomous species and subspecies. The best rule is to leave all snakes alone, give them a wide berth as you hike past, and make sure any hiking companions (including dogs) do the same.

When hiking, stick to well-used trails and wear over-the-ankle boots and loose-fitting long pants. Do not step or put your hands beyond your range of detailed visibility and avoid wandering around in the dark. Step *onto* logs and rocks, never *over* them, and be especially careful when climbing rocks. Always avoid walking through dense brush or willow thickets.

TICKS Ticks are often found on brush and tall grass, where they seem to be waiting to hitch a ride on a warm-blooded passerby. Adult ticks are most active April into May and again October into November. Among the varieties of ticks, the black-legged tick,

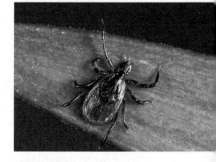

DEER TICK
Jim Gathany/Centers for Disease Control and Prevention (public domain)

commonly called the deer tick, is the primary carrier of Lyme disease. Wear light-colored clothing, making it easier for you to spot ticks before they migrate to your skin. At the end of the hike, visually check your hair, back of neck, armpits, and socks. During your posthike shower, take a moment to do a more complete body check. For ticks that are already embedded, removal with tweezers is best. Use disinfectant solution on the wound.

Hunting

Several rules, regulations, and licenses govern various hunting types and related seasons. Though there are generally no problems, hikers may wish to forgo their trips during the big-game seasons, when the woods suddenly seem filled with orange and camouflage. Hunting is popular in the Upstate, so be sure to check with the South Carolina Department of Natural Resources for specific dates for deer, dove, bear, and turkey hunting; visit dnr.sc.gov.

Regulations

Trail regulations in the Upstate of South Carolina vary depending on where the trail is located. In state parks, always follow posted rules and regulations. For other areas where regulations are not apparent, always use proper trail etiquette and never remove plants or threaten or harass wildlife.

Trail Etiquette

Always treat the trail, wildlife, and fellow hikers with respect. Here are some reminders.

★ *Plan ahead to be self-sufficient at all times.* For example, carry necessary supplies for changes in weather or other conditions. A well-planned trip brings satisfaction to you and to others.

★ *Hike on open trails only.*

★ *Respect trail and road closures.* In seasons or construction areas where road or trail closures may be a possibility, use the website addresses or phone numbers shown in the "Contacts" line for each of this guidebook's hikes to check conditions prior to heading out for your hike. Do not attempt to circumvent such closures.

★ *Avoid trespassing on private land, and obtain all permits and authorization as required.* Also, leave gates as you found them or as directed by signage.

★ *Be courteous to other hikers,* cyclists, equestrians, and others you encounter on the trails.

★ *Never spook wild animals or pets.* An unannounced approach, a sudden movement, or a loud noise startles most animals. A surprised animal can be dangerous to you, to others, and to itself. Give animals plenty of space.

★ *Observe the yield signs around the region's trailheads and backcountry.* Typically, they advise hikers to yield to horses, and bikers to yield to both horses and hikers. On hills, by common courtesy, hikers and bikers yield to any uphill traffic. When encountering mounted riders or horse packers, hikers can courteously step off the trail, on the downhill side if possible. If the horse can see and hear you, calmly greet the riders before they reach you and do not dart behind trees. Also resist the urge to pet horses unless you are invited to do so.

★ *Stay on the existing trail and do not blaze any new trails.*

★ *Be sure to pack out what you pack in, leaving only your footprints.* No one likes to see the trash someone else has left behind.

Tips on Enjoying Hiking in the Upstate

The Upstate of South Carolina is a diverse geographical wonderland. But before embarking on your adventure for any hike in this book, be sure to read the entire entry carefully. Make sure to allow for sufficient driving times and daylight hours, especially in the winter. It is very important during our hot southern days to bring *lots* of water, sunscreen, and bug repellent. Really, don't leave home without these things—I can't stress this enough. Most of all, take your time and enjoy your surroundings instead of hurrying through the hike just to say, "I did it." While the feeling of a completed hike does signify accomplishment, it's also important to enjoy the trees, flowers, waterfalls, mountains, and creeks that make up our great region.

Anderson and Oconee Counties (Hikes 1–6)

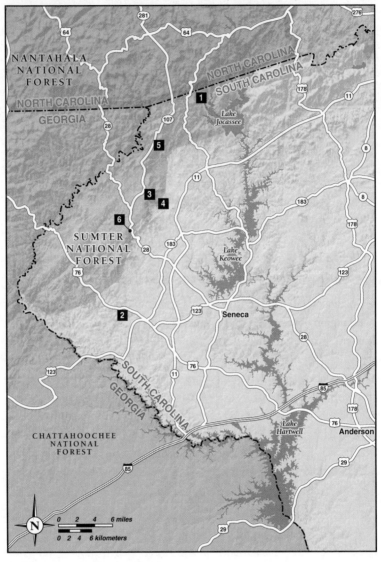

Anderson and Oconee Counties

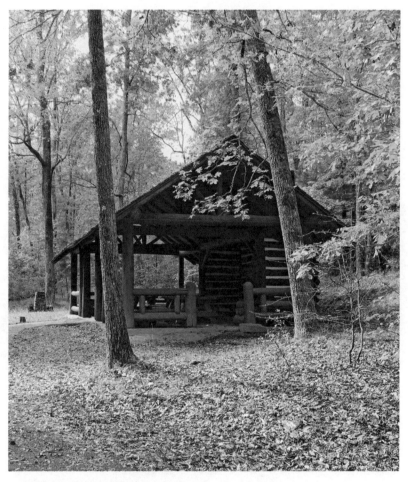

PICNIC SHELTER AT YELLOW BRANCH FALLS *(See Hike 6, page 40.)*

Bad Creek: Lower Whitewater Falls Trail

SCENERY: ★★★★★
TRAIL CONDITION: ★★★
CHILDREN: ★★★
DIFFICULTY: ★★★
SOLITUDE: ★★★

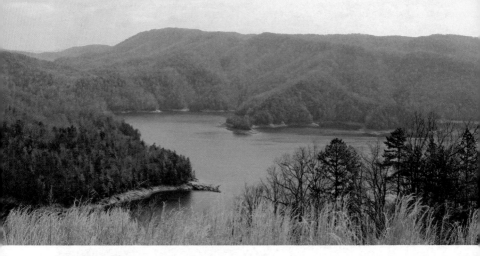

LAKE JOCASSEE

TRAILHEAD GPS COORDINATES: N35° 00.744' W82° 59.950'

DISTANCE & CONFIGURATION: 5.4-mile out-and-back

HIKING TIME: 4 hours

HIGHLIGHTS: Spectacular waterfall, great views of Lake Jocassee and mountains

ELEVATION: 1,959' at trailhead to 2,159' at the top of the hill after the dirt road

ACCESS: Daily, sunrise–sunset; free

MAPS: South Carolina Department of Natural Resources

FACILITIES: Portable restrooms at trailhead

WHEELCHAIR ACCESS: None

COMMENTS: Be sure to drive up to the visitors' overlook for great views of Lake Jocassee and the surrounding mountains.

CONTACT: Duke Energy, 800-443-5193, duke-energy.com/Energy-Education/Energy-Centers-and-Programs/Outdoor-Classroom-at-Bad-Creek-Hydro-Station

Overview

As you enter through the electric-fenced gate, you get the feeling that you're trespassing into some top-secret facility. That's somewhat true. Duke Energy owns this site, and it's home to the company's largest hydroelectric station. That installation includes Lake Jocassee's 7,500 acres, another 375-acre upper reservoir, and an underground tunnel system and powerhouse. Thus, security is warranted, but they also keep the grounds free and open to the public year-round. Bad Creek also serves as a trailhead for the 80-mile-long Foothills Trail and provides access to the Whitewater River, one of South Carolina's best trout streams.

Route Details

Start at the Bad Creek Foothills Trail Access at the parking lot and follow the blue trail blazes toward the Lower Whitewater Falls Overlook. Whitewater Falls is a series of six cascades in North and South Carolina, making up the highest cluster of falls in the eastern United States. Upper Whitewater Falls in North Carolina is the most popular, but South Carolina's Lower Whitewater Falls is just as spectacular and a great hike.

As you start on the trail, you'll immediately begin uphill, to the right, following alongside a concrete drainage ditch that is about a foot deep. The ditch ends at the top of the hill as the trail turns to the left and begins crossing through a flat meadow area. Old-growth timber trees, wildflowers (in spring), and tall grasses blow in the wind as you catch glimpses of Lake Jocassee to the right. When you come to the treeline, you enter the forest and immediately begin uphill again with wooden stairs to assist.

The trail curves before it begins to descend. The path is well marked and decent aside from tree roots encroaching upon it. Wild turkeys are a common sighting, and along the trail, pine needles drop from the many trees above. The trail continues to descend—but not too dramatically—as it winds around. Soon you will hear rushing water before you come to three more sets of wooden stairs and begin a steeper descent.

You move closer and closer to the sound of water as the path levels out and becomes a bit wider. Tall white pine and hemlock trees still surround you as you begin to follow alongside the Whitewater River. A set of double bridges cross the river. Once across you will see signs for Coon Branch Natural Area, 1.2 miles ahead, and the Upper Falls Parking Area, 1.7 miles farther. Follow the blue blazes across the bridges.

Bad Creek: Lower Whitewater Falls Trail

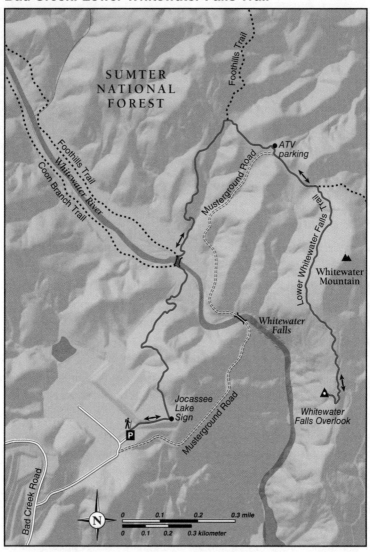

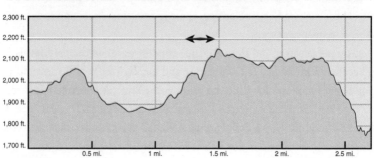

Across the double bridges is another set of signs, and this is where the Foothills Trail branches off. To the left, the trail leads to North Carolina and Oconee State Park (page 27). Follow the trail signs straight ahead, still following the blue blazes. The path is fairly wide and flat here as you cross over a small footbridge. You'll begin walking alongside a small stream as you start to ascend until the path turns toward the left and away from the stream. The trail continues sharply uphill until you reach the crest of Round Mountain Gap. You've hiked about 1.5 miles so far. Here the trail levels out as you walk along the top of the ridge. The sound of the water becomes fainter as the forest gets quiet and you can only hear the wind in the trees. Grassy Knob and other mountains surround you. The trail narrows again as you begin uphill and reach another set of signs. To the left are both the Thompson and Toxaway Rivers. At 0.9 mile straight ahead and to the right is the Lower Whitewater Falls Overlook. Stay on the trail to the overlook, continuing to follow the blue blazes.

The trail leads you uphill for just a short distance until the path widens and you begin a gradual descent. You'll come to a gravel area and dirt road, which is the ATV parking area. Yes, ATVs are allowed here, as is hunting in the Wildlife Management Area lands at nearby Musterground Mountain. Walk through this area, still following the blue blazes, as you now begin walking on a dirt and gravel roadway.

After following the road for a short distance, you'll see the trail to the right and begin immediately uphill with some wooden stairs. You'll continue slightly uphill as you follow alongside a wooded ridge. Through the trees, you'll enjoy views of other mountains. The trail levels out somewhat as you begin to hear the waterfall. As the trail curves around, it begins to descend, starting gradually, then becoming a little steeper. When you reach a set of wooden stairs, you can see glimpses of Lake Jocassee through the trees. The trail continues a steep descent until it ends at the Whitewater Falls Overlook area. Its viewing deck provides a panorama of the majestic 200-foot waterfall in the distance. After resting and enjoying the view, turn around and return the same way.

Nearby Attractions

Bad Creek also offers an outdoor classroom where students can learn about the environment and how Duke Energy generates electricity. The site is in a clearing with tables and benches and two nature trails for students and teachers to experience the region's ecosystems and wildlife. **Devils Fork State Park** is nearby, offering public access to the lake. Boating, swimming, fishing, and kayaking are all available.

Directions

From downtown Easley, head north on US 178 to SC 11. Turn north onto Whitewater Falls Road (SC 130) for 5.8 miles, then turn right onto Bad Creek Road. Go through the gate entrance at Duke Power's Bad Creek Hydroelectric Station and follow signs to the Foothills Trail Parking Area.

LOWER WHITEWATER FALLS FROM THE OVERLOOK

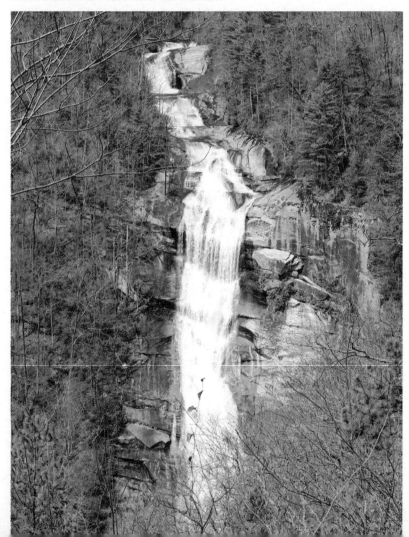

2 # Chau Ram County Park

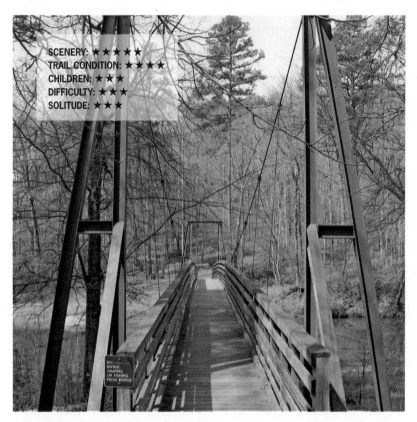

SCENERY: ★★★★★
TRAIL CONDITION: ★★★★
CHILDREN: ★★★
DIFFICULTY: ★★★
SOLITUDE: ★★★

THE LARGEST SUSPENSION BRIDGE IN OCONEE COUNTY IS AT CHAU RAM COUNTY PARK.

TRAILHEAD GPS COORDINATES: N34° 40.921' W83° 08.749'

DISTANCE & CONFIGURATION: 1.8-mile balloon

HIKING TIME: 2.25 hours

HIGHLIGHTS: Several waterfalls

ELEVATION: 504' at trailhead to 888' at peak, where the yellow and blue trails meet

ACCESS: Daily, 7 a.m.–sunset; park closes mid-November–February; $3 parking fee per vehicle

MAPS: None

FACILITIES: Four picnic shelters (one with a large outdoor fireplace), restrooms, kayaking facilities, playground, 26 campsites

WHEELCHAIR ACCESS: Not on the trails, only at picnic areas

COMMENTS: No alcoholic beverages allowed in the park; no lifeguards, so swim at your own risk

CONTACT: Chau Ram County Park, 864-647-9286, experienceoconee.com/parks/chau-ram-park

Chau Ram County Park

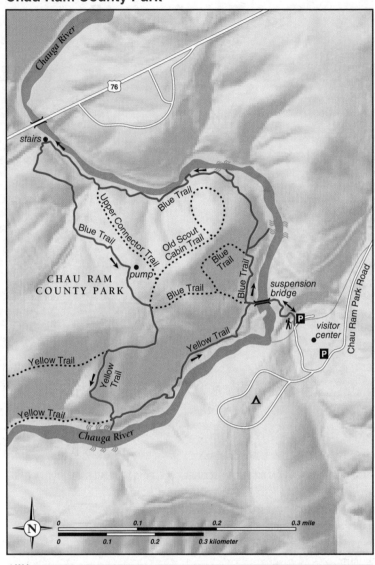

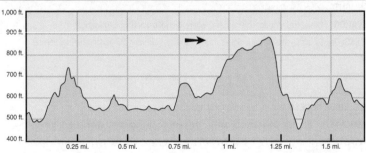

Overview

This park is considered one of Oconee County's best-kept secrets. It's so hidden away in Westminster that even some locals don't know the park exists. This little gem offers waterfalls; sandy beaches with water access for swimming; and four major sets of rapids for kayaking, canoeing, and tubing. Just off the parking lot is the 40-foot Ramsey Falls. There are several other waterfalls downstream.

Route Details

Begin this hike at the lower parking area by Ramsey Falls. Cross the metal-and-wood bridge traversing Ramsey Creek and take the paved pathway up and to the left. Head west to cross the largest suspension bridge in Oconee County, taking you over the Chauga River. A beach area to the right, just before the bridge, has picnic tables and trash cans, making it a great prehike picnic spot.

After crossing the suspension bridge, take the blue loop trail toward the right. The dirt pathway is well marked, and you'll be following alongside the Chauga River. The noise from the pump house across the river can be loud, but it provides a glimpse into how the City of Westminster uses the river as a water-intake area. The pump house also generates rapids—popular with kayakers.

Continuing on the blue trail, you cross a small wooden bridge and another small waterfall just beyond the pump house. A small spur to the right takes you a little closer to the falls. After taking a photo of the falls, come back and continue to the right as you immediately begin a steep climb, still following the blue trail.

The narrow trail follows along the side of the mountain as you ascend farther above the river, gaining a bird's-eye view of the waterfall you just passed. The trail begins to level out, and as you continue along the path, the sound of the pump house fades as you come upon the next waterfall and set of rapids. Kayaking, tubing, and canoeing are allowed on the river, and if you're lucky, on a nice day you can watch the brave souls navigate the rocky waters.

As the trail continues, you leave the rapids behind as the river widens and deepens as you traverse rocks and boulders. The trail goes steeply uphill here and then back down, still following alongside the Chauga River. Without the sounds of rapids and waterfalls you can hear the road noise from nearby US 76. The trail becomes very narrow in spots, so be careful of your footing.

You'll come to a fork in the trail. This is where the Upper Connector Trail (with double red blazes) splits off to the left. This is a shortcut, so if you want a shorter hike, you can take this path back as it cuts through and meets back up with the blue trail. If you're ready to forge ahead—you've gone a little more than 0.5 mile at this point—stay on the blue trail to the right. Just before you go under the US 76 Bridge, a set of 40 wooden stairs leads you up and away from the river.

The trail continues steeply up until you are at the top of the hill and higher than the adjacent highway. At the top of the hill, a trail sign indicates that the blue trail is to the left. Continue following the blue trail. The path is wide and levels out at the top for a short distance until it goes steeply downhill and then uphill again. You're walking through the forest now with the river far in the distance, and though you can still hear traffic sounds, they become fainter the farther into the trees you get.

Continue on the blue trail as it goes to the right. About 1 mile into the hike, a Boy Scout camp clearing to the left offers an old hand-crank water pump and some benches. Soon you arrive at a junction of several paths. Take the yellow path to the right. Again, other paths such as the blue, red, and double red can be taken back for a shorter hike.

As the trail curves and begins to climb slightly uphill, you once again hear the rushing waters from the river below, even though it is not yet in sight. As the trail begins a slightly steep descent, the river once again comes into view. The trail comes to the edge of the river, where there's another small waterfall. Several large, flat boulders here make it the perfect spot for a picnic lunch or sunbathing, or just a nice place to sit next to the rushing water.

The narrow, mostly flat path turns toward the left as the trail takes you to yet another waterfall. You walk along large flat rocks on this part of the trail, following alongside the Chauga River. When you come to the suspension bridge, you've completed the loop portion of the trail. Pass back over the suspension bridge to return to the parking lot, completing the hike.

Nearby Attractions

The campground here is often used as a base for rafting on the nearby **Chattooga River**.

Directions

Drive west on US 76 from Westminster. Keep right at the fork with US 123. Go 2.5 miles to Chau Ram Park Road and turn left. The park entrance is at the end of the road. Follow the park road loop to the lower-level parking area.

Oconee State Park: Old Waterwheel Trail

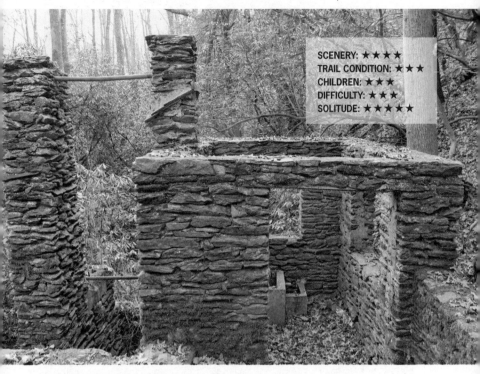

SCENERY: ★ ★ ★ ★
TRAIL CONDITION: ★ ★ ★
CHILDREN: ★ ★ ★
DIFFICULTY: ★ ★ ★
SOLITUDE: ★ ★ ★ ★

THIS OLD WATERWHEEL PUMPED WATER TO THE CCC CAMP IN THE 1940S.

TRAILHEAD GPS COORDINATES: N34° 51.813' W83° 05.882'

DISTANCE & CONFIGURATION: 1.7-mile loop

HIKING TIME: 1.5 hours

HIGHLIGHTS: Seclusion, historic waterwheel, a bamboo forest of switch cane (*Arundinaria*)

ELEVATION: 1,741' at trailhead to 1,847' about 0.5 mile into hike

ACCESS: Sunday–Thursday, 7 a.m.–7 p.m.; Friday–Saturday 7 a.m.–9 p.m. Daylight saving time: daily, 7 a.m.–9 p.m. $5 for age 16 and older; $3.25 for SC seniors; $3 for children ages 6–15; free for age 5 and younger

MAPS: USGS *Oconee State Park*, South Carolina State Parks

FACILITIES: Restrooms and picnic tables in the campground area; none at the trailhead

WHEELCHAIR ACCESS: None

COMMENTS: It's possible to take this trail to the Oconee Connector Trail and connect with Oconee Station.

CONTACT: 864-638-5353, southcarolinaparks.com/oconee

Oconee State Park: Old Waterwheel Trail

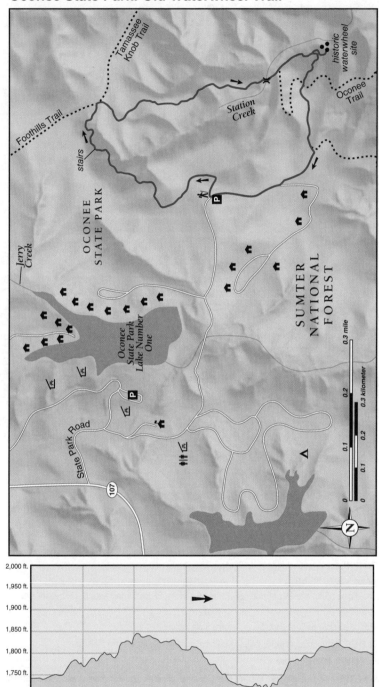

Overview

This trail offers magnificent views and a great deal of solitude in addition to viewing a piece of history. The old waterwheel was used in the early 1900s to pump water to the rest of the camp. This park is a camper's paradise, with 139 campsites, 15 walk-in tent sites, and 19 cabins available for rental. It's also an access point for the Foothills Trail (an 80-mile wilderness trail) and part of the Blue Ridge Escarpment. The park has several other trails available for hiking.

Route Details

Oconee State Park was developed by the Civilian Conservation Corps (CCC) as part of the New Deal program initiated by President Franklin D. Roosevelt during the Great Depression. Several of the buildings crafted by the CCC in the 1930s are still in use at this park.

The trailhead begins across the street from the Foothills Trail parking area. At the trailhead a large sign for the Foothills Trail points to the left. Ignore that and take the trail to the right, marked by a small sign on a tree. The path begins with a gradual descent through a hardwood forest. Continue walking and follow the signs that read OWT (for Old Waterwheel Trail) to the left.

As soon as you make the turn, you will head uphill. The trees turn to oak and pine, with numerous pine needles littering the dirt pathway. As the trail winds around, you begin a slight descent until the path evens out somewhat as you walk along the inside of a punch bowl with a ravine to your right and a hill to your left. The trail is well marked as you continue to follow the orange and white trail signs.

As the trail leads downhill again it continues to wind through the forest. It's super quiet here, with only the crickets chirping and the occasional airplane crossing the sky above you. No matter the time of year, large trees may have fallen, and you may have to make your way over them. Continue along the side of the ravine as it gets deeper, still heading downhill.

The dirt path is narrow and littered with leaves and pine needles. As you round the next corner, you immediately head steeply uphill with a few logs placed as makeshift stairs. You've hiked about 0.4 mile so far. Continue along the top of the rim before heading steeply downhill again. Another uphill climb and several switchbacks later land you in the middle of a fairly level switch cane forest.

The trail here is overgrown in some sections but is cut back enough that you won't lose your way. Continue through the grove of switch cane as the trees get thicker and you begin to hear the trickling of water in the distance. This only lasts for a moment, though, as you veer left and begin another gradual descent. Continue along the top of the mountain this time with a ravine to your left. As you travel farther downhill, another ravine appears on your right. As the ravine on the left gets deeper, the one on the right slowly fades away.

When you come to a small stream you will notice a wooden plank placed across it as a bridge. Follow across the stream as you come to two more moss-covered footbridges. You'll now be walking with the stream on your left and at the bottom of the ravine. You are deep in the forest with hills surrounding you on both sides. It is very still and quiet, without even birds to break the silence.

You'll soon come to a connector sign (approximately 1.2 miles in) that reads WATERWHEEL SITE. Take this path about 50 feet to view the old waterwheel that was used as an overshot wheel to power a piston that pumped water for the CCC camp in the 1940s. Stone pillars and portions of the waterwheel house are all that remain here now.

When you're ready to continue, return to the waterwheel site sign and continue on the trail to the right; it heads steeply uphill with log ties acting as stairs. At the top you come to a fork. To the left is the Oconee Trail (this would take you to Oconee Station), but you want to continue straight ahead toward the sign that says Oconee Park. Here you pick up the green Oconee Trail signs. At the next fork turn right to walk along the old wagon trail. This section of trail is much wider and more level than what you have been following. When you come to the road, follow it a short distance back to the parking lot and trailhead.

Nearby Attractions

In addition to camping, the park has two lakes stocked with bass, catfish, and trout. The park also has pedal boats, johnboats, and canoes available for rental. There's even a playground and minigolf course for the kids. From Memorial Day until Labor Day, the park has bluegrass music and square dancing on Friday nights.

Directions

From I-85 take Exit 1 to SC 11 toward Walhalla. Go approximately 10 miles and then turn right onto SC 107. The park will be about 2 miles on the right.

Oconee Station: Interpretive Nature Trail and Station Cove Trail

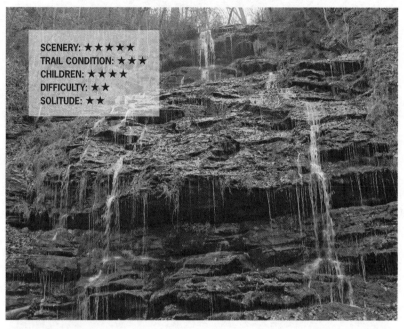

SCENERY: ★ ★ ★ ★ ★
TRAIL CONDITION: ★ ★ ★
CHILDREN: ★ ★ ★ ★
DIFFICULTY: ★ ★
SOLITUDE: ★ ★

STATION COVE FALLS

TRAILHEAD GPS COORDINATES: N34° 50.793' W83° 04.206'

DISTANCE & CONFIGURATION: 3.1-mile balloon

HIKING TIME: 2.25 hours

HIGHLIGHTS: Historic homes, Station Cove Falls, fishing pond

ELEVATION: 1,161' at beginning trailhead to 1,421' at Station Cove Trailhead

ACCESS: Daily, 9 a.m.–6 p.m.; free. Guided tours are offered on some weekends; times vary.

MAPS: USGS *Oconee Station*, South Carolina State Parks

FACILITIES: Restrooms and picnic area at the ranger station

WHEELCHAIR ACCESS: None

COMMENTS: It's possible to take this trail to the Oconee Connector Trail and connect with Oconee State Park. It's a strenuous 4-mile trail with an 800-foot elevation change, so be prepared if you decide to do this. This hike combines two trails—an interpretive nature trail and Station Cove Falls Trail. Station Cove Falls Trail is much busier than the nature trail.

CONTACT: 864-638-0079, southcarolinaparks.com/oconee-station

Oconee Station: Interpretive Nature Trail & Station Cove Trail

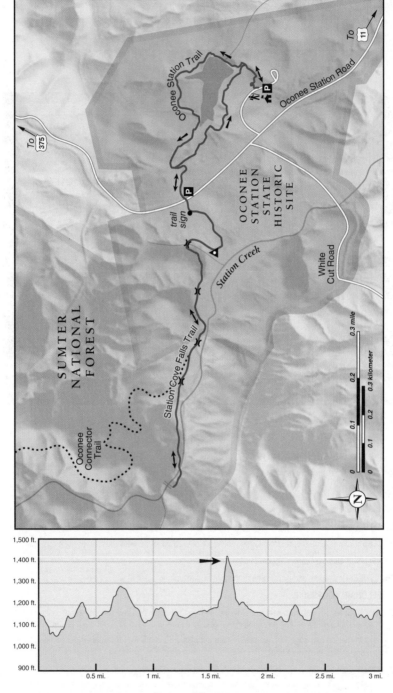

Overview

Here you get a dose of history before combining an interpretive nature trail in the Sumter National Forest and a trail leading to Station Cove Falls. Originally a military compound and later a trading post, Oconee Station State Historic Site gives a glimpse into what life was like in the 1700 and 1800s. The stone block-house, called the Station House, was used as an outpost by the South Carolina militia from 1792 until 1799. The larger William Richards House (named for the Irish immigrant who built the house) served as a family home from 1805 until the park service acquired the land in 1976.

Route Details

Begin at the ranger station and parking lot. Depending on timing, tour the homes first or after you return from your hike. These two structures were located on the front lines of the Revolutionary War and served as a military compound against attack from the Cherokee and Creek Indians.

The trail begins down and across the road from the historic homes. Begin at the sign that reads NATURE TRAIL/POND/FALLS as you go downhill through the trees. Just before the pond you will come to another sign that reads FALLS TO YOUR LEFT. Stay on the trail to your right, as you will go around the pond and still end up at the waterfall, making for a nicer and longer hike. As you get to the fishing pond, continue on the straight and narrow path. The pond is serene and still— it's hard to believe there are a lot of fish swimming beneath the blue-green water.

When you get to the green box at the pond, the trail seems to turn to the right, but it doesn't. Continue straight ahead as the dirt pathway becomes a little harder to follow. As long as you are following along the pond here, you're on the right path. Once you reach the other side of the pond, you will cross over the pond, heading west. There are typically a lot of downed trees in this area, but it's very quiet as you listen to the wind with only the occasional sounds of the station in the background.

You'll soon head downhill, and the pond once again comes into view. Here the trail really levels out and becomes much wider as you walk along a small creek. Soon the path leads away from the pond again and is dotted with many ferns and rich hardwood trees. Once you reach another sign that reads FALLS, follow this trail up and to the right. Fortunately, this steep ascent has wooden stairs to assist. As you turn right again, the trail is marked by a small silver sign on a tree.

At the top of the stairs, there is a road with a small parking area. Cross the road and you will be at the Station Cove Falls Trailhead. If you wanted a much shorter hike, you could park here and just do the Station Cove Falls Trail, which is about 0.9 mile from this point.

The first portion of this trail is part of the Palmetto Trail. The path is fairly easy and wide here. As you continue walking you will come to a bench that overlooks the landscape below. Continue meandering through the forest until you get to a small bridge over an almost nonexistent creek. The trail keeps going, with a ravine on one side and a hill on the other, as it narrows a little.

As you cross a couple more bridges over another small creek, the path stays fairly level. After crossing a fourth bridge, you will come to a sign and a fence. This is where you could take the Oconee Connector Trail that leads to Oconee State Park.

Continue on the trail to the left toward the waterfall. The falls are about 300 feet from this point. A small stream will be on your left as you continue to a stone staircase that leads across the stream and up to the falls. The falls are a nice 70-foot cascade over several rocks jutting out. Several smaller flat rocks make a nice place to sit and relax.

When you are ready to head back (you've trekked about 1.7 miles), continue on the same trail until you cross back over the roadway. When you come to another falls sign, turn right as the trail leads downhill and back to the ranger station and parking lot.

Nearby Attractions

The 4-acre fishing pond is stocked with bluegill and largemouth bass. The **Palmetto Trail,** with access from the Station Cove Trail, is a challenging and popular mountain bike trail. See page 78 for a hike thst incorporates a section of the Palmetto Trail.

Directions

From I-85 South, take Exit 19B (SC 28) toward Clemson. Go about 26 miles to the SC 11 ramp and turn right onto SC 11. Drive about 6 miles and turn left onto Oconee Station Road. The park entrance will be in 2 miles.

Winding Stairs Trail

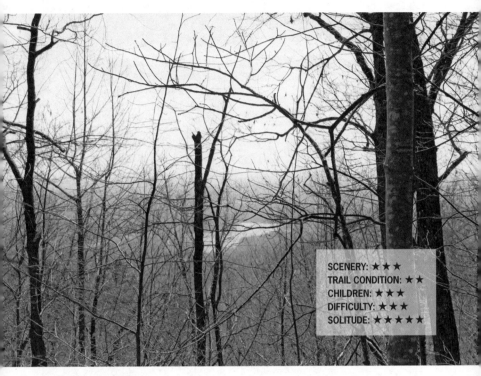

SCENERY: ★ ★ ★
TRAIL CONDITION: ★ ★
CHILDREN: ★ ★ ★
DIFFICULTY: ★ ★ ★
SOLITUDE: ★ ★ ★ ★ ★

VIEWS OF LAKE CHEOHEE

TRAILHEAD GPS COORDINATES: N34° 56.479' W83° 05.393' (northern trailhead),
N34° 55.336' W83° 04.650' (southern trailhead)

DISTANCE & CONFIGURATION: 7.2-mile out-and-back or 3.6-mile point-to-point

HIKING TIME: 4.5 hours

HIGHLIGHTS: Tranquility, mountain views, two waterfalls, challenging elevation change

ELEVATION: 2,257' at trailhead to 2,336' at peak (near beginning of hike) and 1,219' at lowest point

ACCESS: Sunrise–sunset; free

MAPS: USFS *Francis Marion and Sumter National Forests*

FACILITIES: There are restroom facilities at nearby Cherry Hill Recreation Area but only during late spring and summer months. Primitive camping is allowed as long as campsites are more than 50' from streams and trails and a quarter mile from roads.

WHEELCHAIR ACCESS: None

COMMENTS: Dogs are allowed on leashes. For an easier, shorter hike, bring two vehicles and park one at the northern trailhead and one at the southern trailhead.

CONTACT: Sumter National Forest, Andrew Pickens Ranger District, 864-638-9568, fs.usda.gov/scnfs

Winding Stalrs Trail

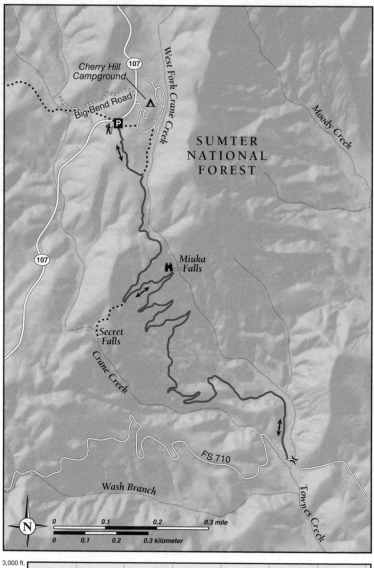

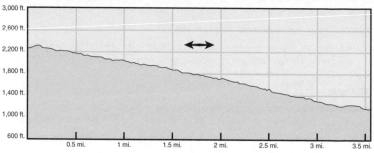

Overview

The South Carolina Trails Program calls this trail "one of the finest beginner trails in northwest South Carolina." Of course, the person who wrote that description must have only hiked the trail downhill. When hiking both out and back, this trail provides a decent workout with more than 1,000 feet in elevation change. Aptly named Winding Stairs for the numerous switchbacks, or natural staircases, the trail also offers great views of two waterfalls and surrounding mountains.

Route Details

Winding Stairs is set in the Andrew Pickens Ranger District of Sumter National Forest. Sumter National Forest comprises almost 371,000 acres in South Carolina, and the Andrew Pickens District is its crown jewel. Located in the mountainous western edge of the state, elevations here range from 800 to 3,400 feet, and the district has numerous waterfalls and hiking trails.

Begin this hike at the northern trailhead parking area. The trailhead and parking can be a little hard to find, but it's just south of the Cherry Hill Recreation Area. There is a small dirt pullout, and the trailhead is marked by a brown pole sign. The trail begins immediately uphill following a narrow dirt pathway as it curves around to the left. You're at the top of the mountain here, walking through a forest filled with white pines, cedars, oaks, and poplars. The ground is littered with leaves and fallen branches, but it's quiet and peaceful, especially during fall and winter.

Soon the trail descends until it levels out somewhat and then resumes downhill again. The trail is not well marked, but the path is still fairly easy to follow. Continue until you reach a fork. To the left is Cherry Hill Recreation Area and to the right is the southern trailhead (3.4 miles from this point). Take the trail to the right.

Follow a level path along West Fork Crane Creek. As you hike notice the canopy of rhododendron trees that provide shade, while the sound of the rushing creek provides solace. As the creek lowers into the valley, the trail widens, and though you can't see the creek anymore, you can still hear the rushing water.

The trail winds around the mountain, and there are some rock outcrops to the left. The creek is even more in the distance now and can barely be heard. As you round the next corner you will enjoy great glimpses through the trees of the surrounding mountains and Lake Cheohee in the valley below. In winter the views are even more amazing.

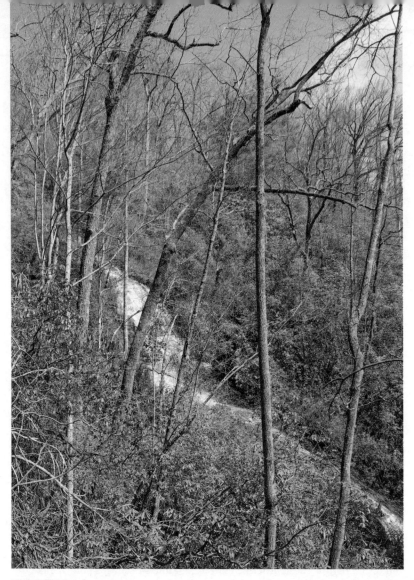

MIUKA FALLS

The pathway narrows again as you continue following the mountain ridge. It's still fairly level here with only a slight descent. But as you continue winding downhill, you'll notice the mountain to the left becoming higher, indicating that you are proceeding downhill at a good pace.

You'll soon come to a turnoff where the trail abruptly veers to the left. This is indicated by a rust-colored trail blaze (one of very few). It isn't easy to spot, so keep an eye out for it. This is where your descent begins to steepen, but with the many switchbacks, it's not too difficult to maneuver.

As you head back in the direction of the creek, you'll pass over a few small runoff areas that can be quite muddy and tricky to traverse. You'll cross over these again and again as both you and the water head downhill.

You'll hear Miuka Falls way before you see it, about 1.3 miles into the hike. A small turnoff to the left provides pretty good views. Again, the path isn't well marked, so be on the lookout. The cascading water billows down about 75 feet over several sets of rocks, making this quite a spectacular waterfall.

After viewing the waterfall, continue on the trail to the right as it proceeds downward with several switchbacks to make the descent less noticeable. There are usually several downed trees to hurdle over, as well as a few small muddy streams to navigate. About two-thirds of the way down (1.9 miles), there is a turnoff to the right. This takes you to Secret Falls, a smaller waterfall. Be careful if you hike to this one, as the path to the waterfall is pretty steep.

As you get near the bottom, you once again hear the rushing creek and follow alongside it. The trail ends at the dirt parking area of the southern trailhead.

If you're doing the hike out-and-back, spend some time at the creek and rest up—the trek back uphill is quite a workout!

Nearby Attractions

Cherry Hill Recreation Area has a 29-site campground with restrooms, showers, and a dump station. However, it's open only during late spring and summer. The **Walhalla State Fish Hatchery** is close by, as is the **Chattooga River.**

Directions

Northern trailhead: Take SC 28 west of Walhalla for about 7.5 miles to SC 107. Turn right and drive 8.8 miles. The trailhead is in a small turnoff parking area on the right, just before you reach the Cherry Hill Recreation Area.

Southern trailhead: Take SC 28 west of Walhalla for about 7.5 miles to SC 107. Go about 5.8 miles and then turn right onto Forest Service Road 710; look for a small FOOTHILLS TRAIL sign marking the turnoff. Drive 2.5 miles on this one-lane gravel road until you reach a small parking area and trailhead on the left, just before the Townes Creek Bridge.

6

Yellow Branch Falls

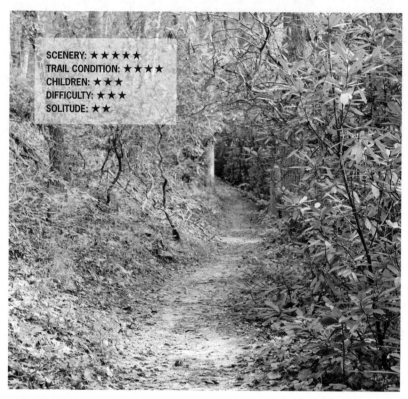

SCENERY: ★ ★ ★ ★ ★
TRAIL CONDITION: ★ ★ ★ ★
CHILDREN: ★ ★ ★
DIFFICULTY: ★ ★ ★
SOLITUDE: ★ ★

YELLOW BRANCH FALLS TRAIL

TRAILHEAD GPS COORDINATES: N34° 48.350' W83° 07.728'

DISTANCE & CONFIGURATION: 3.4-mile out-and-back

HIKING TIME: 2.5 hours

HIGHLIGHTS: 50-foot waterfall at hike's end

ELEVATION: 1,473' at trailhead to 1,530' about 0.1 mile into the hike

ACCESS: Daily, 6 a.m.–10 p.m.; free

MAPS: USFS *Sumter National Forest*

FACILITIES: Picnic tables and a wood shelter with huge rock fireplace; restroom at lower loop parking lot

WHEELCHAIR ACCESS: Only to the shelter and restroom, not on the trail

COMMENTS: Dogs are allowed but must be leashed. Wear sturdy shoes, especially if the ground is wet and slippery, as you will be edging along some deep ravines. There are two parking areas, a lower and an upper lot; park in the lower area if spaces are available.

CONTACT: Sumter National Forest, Andrew Pickens Ranger District, 864-638-9568, fs.usda.gov/scnfs

Overview

This moderate hiking trail in the Sumter National Forest is beautiful any time of year, but the waterfall at the end of the hike is best after a good rain. Even when the trail and picnic area are crowded on a nice weekend, the tall pine and hardwood trees make it feel secluded.

Route Details

Sumter National Forest was designated a national forest in 1936 and has more than 371,000 acres. Yellow Branch Falls is part of the Andrew Pickens Ranger District, which covers the western edge of South Carolina. The mountainous district is named for Andrew Pickens, who served as a commander in the rebel militia during the American Revolutionary War and the Cherokee War of 1760–1761, and in the South Carolina General Assembly. Pickens was instrumental in the Treaty of Hopewell with the Cherokee and was the first member of the United States Congress from the Pendleton District. Pickens built a plantation in the former village of Tamassee, which is located in the Andrew Pickens Ranger District. Elevations in the area range from 800 to more than 3,400 feet, and the forest features a variety of terrain, activities, and other outdoor opportunities.

There are actually two trails at Yellow Branch. The first is a short nature trail (0.4-mile loop trail); the second is the longer out-and-back Yellow Branch Falls Trail. Both begin at the same point, which can be tricky to find as it is poorly marked. Begin to the left of the lower picnic area, toward the road. The trail starts off partially paved with asphalt and rock, as the first section is the Yellow Branch Nature Trail. When you hear the murmur of the nearby creek, turn toward the right. The trail quickly turns to dirt and travels slightly downhill while following a small creek on the left. It feels secluded here with tall oak, gum, and pine trees on both sides. Rhododendron and mountain laurel dot the banks of the small streams you will encounter along the way.

Natural stepping stones enable you to cross over the small creek, which will now be on your right side as you continue the slight descent and the trail begins to curve around. Cross the creek twice more before coming to a fork. Head right, on the trail marked with a sign that reads TO YELLOW BRANCH FALLS TRAIL. Soon you come to a bridge that takes you across the creek again. The trail here is fairly level but be careful of the numerous tree roots that are trying to push out of the ground. When you get to the creek again, cross to the left and continue on the pathway.

Yellow Branch Falls

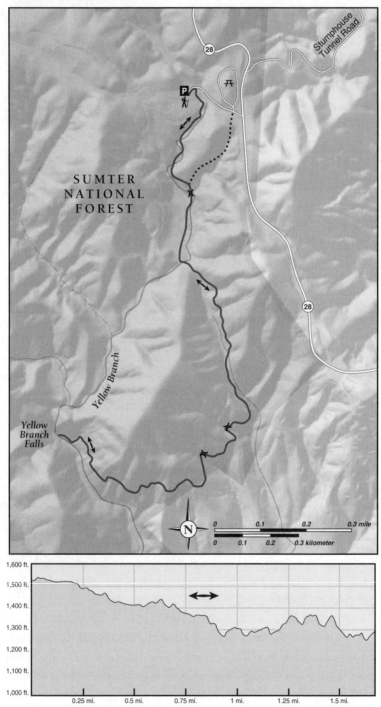

The trail begins to narrow and get muddier (especially if it's been raining recently) as you walk along a deep ravine. Be careful of your footing and use extra caution here. You'll begin to pick up sounds of a small trickle from another stream, but it's very faint, as it's located at the bottom of the ravine. Elevation changes are apparent as you make your way along the trail. At times you can hear cars passing on the roadway nearby, but mostly it's quiet and tranquil. During winter, when the trees are bare, you can catch glimpses of the town of Walhalla as you make your way along the trail.

Pretty soon you come to another footbridge, and depending on the time of year, it may or may not have water running under it. Continue walking along the left side of the ravine until you come to another bridge, at which point you begin a moderately steep uphill trek, still along the ravine.

You can hear the waterfall before you see it as you begin your descent, still hugging the ravine. Soon you will come upon the 50-foot waterfall cascade at 1.7 miles into the hike. While these falls are not as tall as others in the Upstate, the number of rocks jutting out and the 75-foot expanse make the falls impressive, with many vertical cascades of water. Take time to enjoy the waterfall before heading back the way you came.

Nearby Attractions

Stumphouse Tunnel is a 1,617-foot-long abandoned railroad tunnel that is one of the most visited sites in South Carolina. It's considered somewhat of an oddity and a monument to pre–Civil War engineering. **Issaqueena Falls** is a 200-foot cascading waterfall named for a woman from a Creek Indian legend. Both are just up the road, less than a mile from Yellow Branch Falls.

Directions

From Walhalla take SC 28 west for about 7 miles. The turnoff to the Yellow Branch Falls parking area will be on your left, marked by a brown SUMTER NATIONAL FOREST sign.

Bonus Hikes in Oconee County

Here are three more hikes to try in Sumter National Forest. **Note:** I haven't hiked these myself; instead, I gathered information from other hikers and online sources.

 ## East Fork Trail

DISTANCE & CONFIGURATION: Approximately 5-mile out-and-back

HIKING TIME: Approximately 3–4 hours

HIGHLIGHTS: Chattooga River

ACCESS: Daily, sunrise–sunset; free

MAPS: USFS *Sumter National Forest*

FACILITIES: Restrooms and water at Walhalla Fish Hatchery; primitive camping allowed along the trail

WHEELCHAIR ACCESS: None

CONTACT: Sumter National Forest, Andrew Pickens Ranger District, 864-638-9568, fs.usda.gov/scnfs

Overview

This easy hike follows alongside the Chattooga River. There are two trailheads, but it's suggested to begin at the Chattooga Picnic Area, adjacent to the Walhalla Fish Hatchery.

To get there: From Walhalla, drive northwest on SC 28 for 7.5 miles and bear right onto SC 107. Drive 12 miles and turn left onto Fish Hatchery Road (Oconee County Road S-325). Continue to the fish hatchery and picnic area. The eastern trailhead is at the bridge.

While you're there check out the only trout hatchery in South Carolina—150,000 pounds of rainbow, brown, and brook trout are raised here each year to stock area streams and lakes.

 ## Riley Moore Falls Trail

DISTANCE & CONFIGURATION: Approximately 1.9-mile out-and-back

HIKING TIME: Approximately 1 hour

HIGHLIGHTS: 100-foot-wide and 12-foot-high waterfall on the Chauga River

ACCESS: Daily, sunrise–sunset; free

MAPS: USFS *Sumter National Forest*

FACILITIES: None

WHEELCHAIR ACCESS: None

COMMENTS: Hikers have indicated online that the logging road leading to the trail can be difficult If it has rained recently and suggest bringing a four-wheel-drive vehicle.

CONTACT: Sumter National Forest, Andrew Pickens Ranger District, 864-638-9568, fs.usda.gov/scnfs

Overview

One of the Upstate's newer trails, Riley Moore Falls Trail offers a moderate hike to a spectacular waterfall. The trail gets its name from Riley Moore, a former mill that was located at the top of the falls.

To get there: From Westminster, drive west 7.5 miles on US 76 and turn right onto Cobb Bridge Road (Oconee County Road S-37). Drive 1.6 miles, then turn left onto Spy Rock Road (gravel Forest Service Road 748). Drive 1.8 miles to FS 748C (on the right) and park by the side of the road. Hike east on FS 748C for 0.3 mile to the trail and hike 0.7 mile to the waterfall.

This hike is near Yellow Branch Falls, Issaqueena Falls, and Stumphouse Tunnel. All could easily be combined into a day-long excursion.

 # Ross Mountain Passage of the Palmetto Trail

DISTANCE & CONFIGURATION: 5-mile point-to-point

HIKING TIME: Not available

HIGHLIGHTS: Connector to Oconee State Park and Oconee Passage

ACCESS: Sunday–Thursday, 7 a.m.–7 p.m., extended to 9 p.m. during daylight saving time; Friday–Saturday, 7 a.m.–9 p.m. Admission required Into Oconee State Park: $6 for age 16 and older; $3.75 for seniors; $3.50 for children ages 6–15; free for age 5 and younger

MAPS: Online at palmettoconservation.org/passage/ross-mountain

FACILITIES: Camping and restrooms available at Oconee State Park

WHEELCHAIR ACCESS: None

CONTACT: Palmetto Conservation Foundation, 803-771-0870, palmettoconservation.org/passage /ross-mountain

Overview

Another newer trail in the Upstate, Ross Mountain Passage connects Oconee State Park to Stumphouse Passage, with a connector to Stumphouse Mountain Bike Park. The trail is located within Sumter National Forest's Andrew Pickens Ranger District.

Oconee State Park offers camping and two lakes stocked with bass, catfish, and trout. Paddleboats, johnboats, and canoes are available for rental. There's also a playground and minigolf course for the kids.

The trailhead is located at 624 State Park Road, Mountain Rest, SC.

Pickens County (Hikes 7–12)

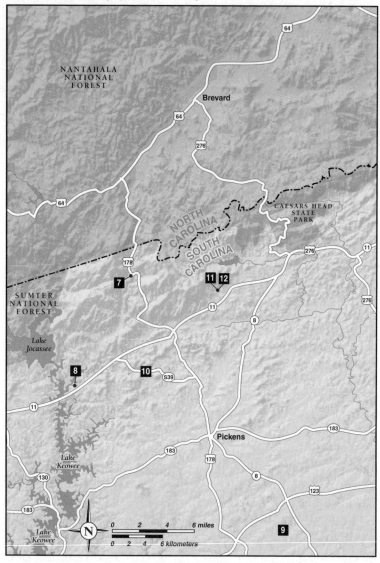

Pickens County

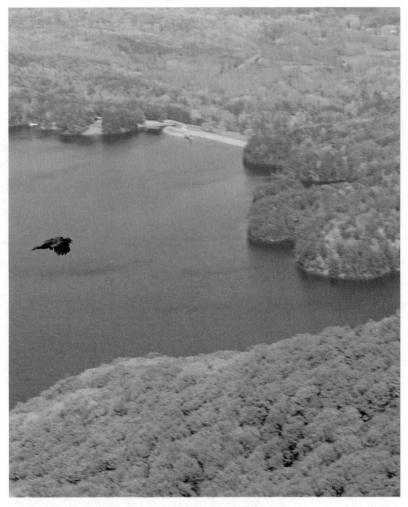

A HAWK FLIES OVER THE WATERSHED AT TABLE ROCK STATE PARK.
(See Hike 12, page 71.)

7

Eastatoe Creek
Heritage Preserve Trail

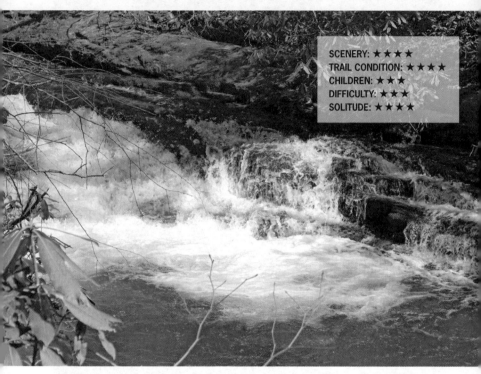

SCENERY: ★ ★ ★ ★
TRAIL CONDITION: ★ ★ ★ ★
CHILDREN: ★ ★ ★
DIFFICULTY: ★ ★ ★
SOLITUDE: ★ ★ ★ ★

EASTATOE CREEK

TRAILHEAD GPS COORDINATES: N35° 02.948' W82° 48.837'

DISTANCE & CONFIGURATION: 6.2-mile out-and-back

HIKING TIME: 4 hours

HIGHLIGHTS: Mountain gorge, two waterfalls, and a stream

ELEVATION: 1,799' at trailhead to 1,951' at peak near the start of the hike

ACCESS: Daily, sunrise–sunset; free

MAPS: South Carolina Department of Natural Resources

FACILITIES: None

WHEELCHAIR ACCESS: None

COMMENTS: Dogs are allowed but must be leashed. Several websites indicate this is a 1.7-mile one-way hike, but that it is incorrect. Also, hunting and fishing are allowed in accordance with WMA regulations. Primitive camping used to be allowed but is now prohibited.

CONTACT: South Carolina Department of Natural Resources, 864-654-6738, dnr.sc.gov

Overview

The Eastatoe Creek Heritage Preserve is located within the Jocassee Gorges, which was named by *National Geographic* as one of "50 of the World's Last Great Places." Jocassee, meaning "place of the lost one" according to Native Americans, was home to several Indian tribes, including the Eastatoe. The 43,000-acre natural area is home to amazing waterfalls and diverse plant life. The Eastatoe Creek Heritage Preserve covers 374 acres, features dramatic rock cliffs and a rainbow trout stream, and is home to three rare ferns.

Route Details

This moderate hiking trail begins at the Foothills Trail parking area and ascends slightly uphill on the gravel road about 500 feet until you get to a turnoff area. Signage here says you are at the right place, the Eastatoe Creek Heritage Preserve. Head to the left past the red barrier gate and begin the trail.

The dirt and gravel path is fairly wide as you begin your journey, following an old logging road. A deep gorge is to the left as you wind around with a mountain on the right. Following the yellow blazes, the trail curves quite a bit but is mostly level. You will have amazing views of nearby Sassafras Mountain, the highest point in South Carolina at 3,533 feet above sea level.

As you bear right, the old logging road you've been following cuts through a small mountain. After this you come to a fork in the trail. Head left, still following the yellow trail blazes and Eastatoe Creek Preserve signs. The trail immediately begins uphill here, hugging the side of the mountain on the left. The dirt pathway becomes a little sandier, and the trail curves toward the left as it begins to level out just a little.

Continue to follow the ridge of the mountaintop as the trail snakes along. You'll begin a slight descent and notice how quiet and peaceful it is here. There are still amazing views of Sassafras Mountain and the surrounding area.

At the next fork in the trail, continue to follow the Eastatoe signs and yellow blazes. The trail ascends until it levels out again and winds around yet another mountain. Depending on recent rainfall, the path can be muddy here, so watch your footing as you listen to the wind whipping through the canyon below.

As the trail narrows slightly, you continue along with the mountain on the right and the gorge to the left. Rock outcrops begin to appear as the path continues downhill. When you get to the LAND AND WATER CONSERVATION sign, the trail abruptly veers left and begins a dramatic descent at 2.3 miles into

Eastatoe Creek Heritage Preserve Trail

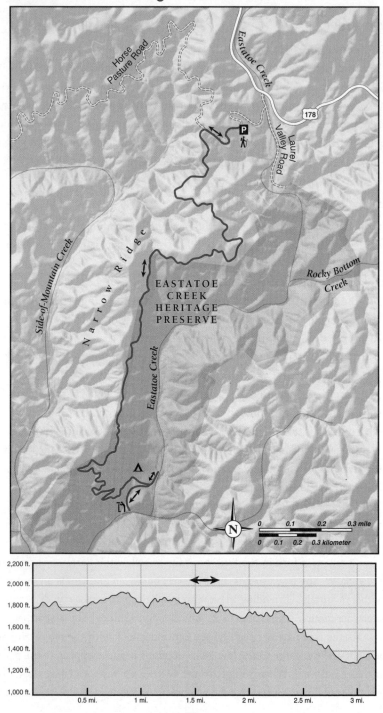

the hike. Eight sets of wooden stairs assist, but it's single file from here; the trail becomes quite narrow as it snakes its way down the mountain.

A few wooden bridges and footbridges provide additional assistance over stream crossings, and several switchbacks aid in the steep descent. The sound of rushing water becomes louder and louder the farther down you go.

When you reach the bottom, you will come to a fork with a sign indicating that the narrows are to the right. Continue on the path to the left, toward Eastatoe Creek and you'll come upon a small but fierce waterfall. Here you can see trout swimming in the stream—this is a popular fishing spot. This part of the trail ends here, so turn around and head back after viewing.

Now take the trail to the right, following the sign that reads the narrows. You'll come to a wooden overlook with great views of Eastatoe Falls, also known as The Narrows, a 60-foot waterfall that tumbles down large rocks and boulders into a series of narrow channels, hence the name. The unusual humidity levels enable three rare tropical fern species to grow here, one of which, the Turnbridge Fern, is not found anywhere else in North America.

Of course, what comes down must go back up, so rest up and then head the 3.1 miles back up the trail.

Nearby Attractions

Access to the Foothills Trail is near the parking area. From here you can hike 8.1 miles to **Laurel Fork Falls** or 61.7 miles to **Oconee State Park.**

Directions

The trail is in Sunset, South Carolina, in Pickens County. From the intersection of US 11 and US 178, go north on US 178 about 7.5 miles. Turn left just after the Eastatoe Creek Bridge, about 1 mile north of the Rock Bottom community. Take the narrow gravel road up to the Foothills parking area.

Keowee-Toxaway State Park: Raven Rock Trail

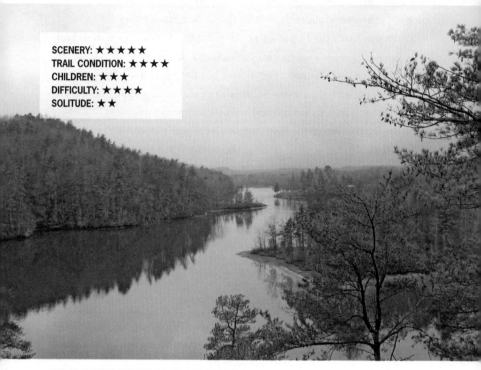

SCENERY: ★★★★★
TRAIL CONDITION: ★★★★
CHILDREN: ★★★
DIFFICULTY: ★★★★
SOLITUDE: ★★

VIEWS OF LAKE KEOWEE FROM RAVEN ROCK

TRAILHEAD GPS COORDINATES: N34° 55.970' W82° 53.123'

DISTANCE & CONFIGURATION: 4.8-mile figure eight (linear/double-loop combination)

HIKING TIME: 4 hours

HIGHLIGHTS: Amazing views of Lake Keowee and the Blue Ridge Mountains, and a natural bridge

ELEVATION: 1,085' at trailhead to 1,193' about 1.5 miles into the hike

ACCESS: Saturday–Thursday, 9 a.m.–6 p.m.; Friday, 9 a.m.–8 p.m. Daylight saving time: daily, 9 a.m.–9 p.m.; free

MAPS: Keowee-Toxaway State Park

FACILITIES: Restrooms and water at visitor center; camping and cabin rentals and a canoe and kayak launch available in the park

WHEELCHAIR ACCESS: At the visitor center but not on the trails

COMMENTS: This park is dog-friendly, with waste disposal bags at the trailhead.

CONTACT: Keowee-Toxaway State Park, 864-868-2605, southcarolinaparks.com/keowee-toxaway

Overview

Keowee-Toxaway State Park is considered the gateway to the 43,000-acre Jocassee Gorges, named by *National Geographic* as one of "50 of the World's Last Great Places." Jocassee Gorges is known for its amazing waterfalls and diverse plant life (including more than 60 species of rare or endangered plants). The trail offers amazing views of and access to Lake Keowee, and traverses land that the Cherokee once inhabited. Views of the Blue Ridge Mountains are stunning, and in springtime, wildflowers line the trail.

Route Details

Beginning at the Jocassee Visitor Center parking area, this hike combines both the Natural Bridge Trail and Raven Rock Trail. Begin by following the trail signs for the Natural Bridge Trail. The pathway starts out as rock and dirt, but the rock disappears at the lower parking lot area. The trail is smooth and well marked as it follows SC 11 for a short while.

The path continues with only a few small ups and downs until you come upon a bench to your right. Here you are still close to the highway and can hear traffic passing by. Directly past the bench, you come to a fork. This is the start of the loop portion of the Natural Bridge Trail. Continue to the right as you make your way downhill for a short distance until the path once again levels out.

As the trail curves around and finally heads away from the road, you come upon a set of stairs before heading downhill again. You will hear rushing water and see a couple of large rocks as you pass by. Now you are walking along a rim with gorges on either side of you. As you continue downhill, the sound of water gets closer, off to your left.

As you continue a steeper descent, the forest gets thicker and seemingly envelops you as the sound of rushing water gets nearer and nearer. You will come to the natural bridge—a nice, wide, slightly angled rock that straddles the stream. There are many huge boulders here, and for the first time you can no longer hear the traffic from the highway, as the flowing stream drowns out any other sounds.

After the bridge, immediately begin uphill before the path turns to the left and evens out a little. Continue to follow alongside the stream for just a short distance until you come to a fork and sign. Proceeding straight would continue on the Natural Bridge Trail, but you should go right on the Raven Rock Trail, at approximately 0.7 mile.

Keowee-Toxaway State Park: Raven Rock Trail

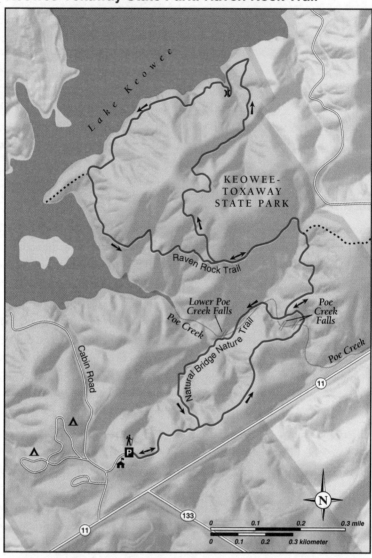

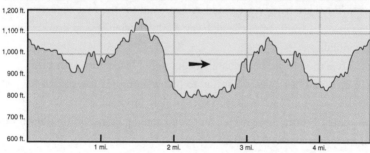

You encounter a few steps as you begin a moderate uphill climb. You are now following the red Raven Rock Trail signs. As you leave the stream below in the distance, you once again hear the sounds from the highway, even though you feel as if you are deep in the forest. As you twist and turn and continue to climb, you will be walking alongside a shallow ravine to the left and a group of rock outcrops forming to your right.

The trail is narrow in spots as you continue with the rock outcrops to the right and the deepening ravine to the left. As you proceed, you will traverse over a couple of small stone runoff bridges and even a rock where a few stone steps have been carved. The trail begins downhill here, and even with the traffic noise you can hear birds chirping.

As the trail continues, you will soon hear the trickle of a small creek before you see a pretty long switchback that, yes, you must do. As you round the bend, begin a slight uphill ascent with the ravine still to the left. A few stone stairs aid your climb along the narrow but well-maintained trail. You pick up the sound of the rushing stream below as you finally lose the sound of the highway again. Pine permeates the air. When you are almost to the top of the hill, after hiking 1.3 miles, you will come to another fork. This begins the loop portion of the Raven Rock Trail. Continue to the right.

At the top, the view is amazing, with the Blue Ridge Mountains in the distance. The path continues uphill with several switchbacks, and you can see the trail that you will soon be following below. As you continue to snake alongside the mountain you once again lose the sound of the stream and pick up the sound of the highway, albeit more in the distance than before. You soon reach the top of the mountain and will see the amazing vistas to the right now instead of the left.

As the trail turns to the left, make your way downhill as you traverse the back side of the mountain. You begin to lose the sound of the stream and the highway and there is only silence. The trail continues to snake down and around the mountain. Be careful if it has rained recently, as the leaf-littered path here can get muddy and slippery.

As you round the corner, you begin to hear the trickle of another small creek and catch glimpses of Lake Keowee to the right. As you get closer to the lake, the trail wraps around and gets close enough to the lake that you could take a dip if you were so inclined. As the trail skirts the edge of Lake Keowee, there will be a small footbridge to cross. The path is fairly level as it continues alongside the lake until you come to a fork. To the right leads to primitive camp-sites down by the lake. Continue on the trail slightly left and straight ahead.

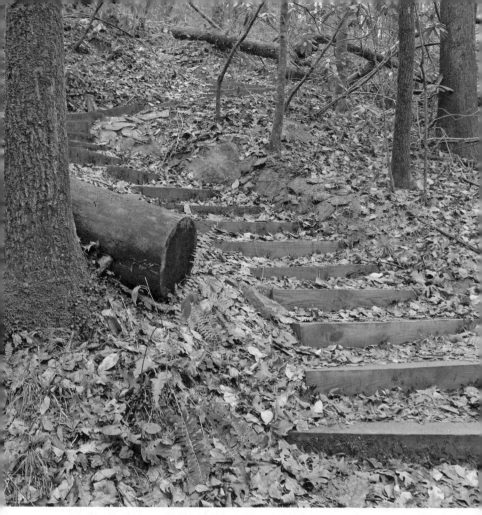

WOODEN STAIRS HELP HIKERS NAVIGATE RAVEN ROCK TRAIL.

Begin climbing, with the lake to your right and the mountain to your left. As you round the next corner you will be at Raven Rock. It's really just a bunch of flat rocks, but it has magnificent views of Lake Keowee. As you make your way farther uphill, the trail begins to take you away from the lake, still hugging the mountain.

You weave around the mountain as you continue climbing uphill. At the top of the mountain you will complete the 1.9 mile Raven Rock loop portion of the hike. Continue on the trail to the right and you'll notice that this is a portion of the same trail that you hiked before. As soon as you reach the top you immediately begin to hear the rushing stream below and traffic in the distance. The trail heads downhill.

As you make your way down the mountain, the rushing stream becomes louder, and on nice days you can hear children playing in the water. Soon you arrive at the fork and loop portion of the Natural Bridge Trail. Take the trail to the right. A set of wooden stairs takes you closer to the creek and a bench at the bottom supplies great views of several waterfalls. It is 0.7 mile from here back to the parking lot. A set of stones serves as a bridge across the rushing creek. You are now following the blue NATURAL BRIDGE TRAIL signs.

The mostly level path continues with just a few ups and downs, with the creek on your right, until you begin a pretty steep uphill climb before the path evens out and begins a steep descent. When you cross a small stream, you go uphill again. The landscape is lusher here than down by the river. You'll soon come to a staircase that assists in the steep climb. As you continue the mostly uphill trek, you begin to turn away from the rushing creek, but you'll still be following along a different, smaller creek. Continue the steep uphill climb until finally you come to the end of the loop portion of the Natural Bridge Trail and the end of the hike.

Nearby Attractions

If you lack time to do the Raven Rock Trail, you can hike the 1.5-mile loop **Natural Bridge Trail**. The **Jocassee Visitor Center** has exhibits and three-dimensional topographical maps on the history of the Jocassee Gorges region and the Cherokee Indians who lived there.

Directions

From I-85 take Exit 40 (SC 153) north for 5 miles. Merge onto US 123 and go north 2.5 miles. US 123 becomes SC 93; continue about 3 miles until you get to SC 8. Continue north for 6 miles. Turn left onto SC 183 and then turn right onto US 178 for 8.5 miles. Turn left onto SC 11 and drive 8.5 miles. Parking will be on the right.

9 Nalley Brown Nature Park: Nalley Trail

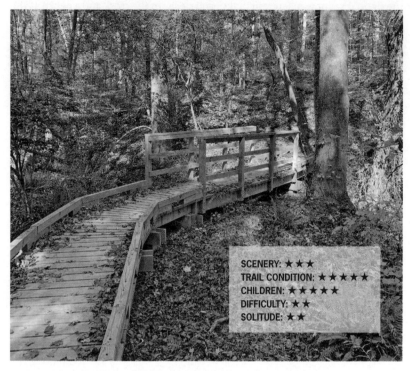

SCENERY: ★ ★ ★
TRAIL CONDITION: ★ ★ ★ ★ ★
CHILDREN: ★ ★ ★ ★ ★
DIFFICULTY: ★ ★
SOLITUDE: ★ ★

WOODEN BRIDGES TRAVERSE WETLANDS AT NALLEY BROWN NATURE PARK.

TRAILHEAD GPS COORDINATES: N34° 47.993' W82° 37.072'

DISTANCE & CONFIGURATION: 1.4-mile loop

HIKING TIME: Approximately an hour

HIGHLIGHTS: Easily located near downtown Easley

ELEVATION: 982' at trailhead to 1019' approximately 1.2 miles into the hike

ACCESS: Daily, sunrise–sunset; free

MAPS: cityofeasley.com/departments/recreation/nalley_brown_nature_park.php

FACILITIES: No restrooms; one shelter and a playground

WHEELCHAIR ACCESS: 1-mile ADA-accessible trail at the park

COMMENTS: This is a great place to come for a quick, after-work hike during the summer.

CONTACT: City of Easley, 864-855-7933, cityofeasley.com/departments/recreation/nalley_brown_nature_park.php

Overview

The newest park in Easley, the 38-acre Nalley Brown Nature Park offers three trails spanning 2.5 miles in an easy-to-get-to urban setting (it's only 3 miles from downtown Easley). Great for an after-work hike or one with kids in tow, the park is named after the Nalley and Brown families who farmed the property and owned it for over 150 years before Catherine Brown Ladnier donated it to the city of Easley in 2001.

Route Details

After parking in the parking lot, which can get full on weekends, start at the trailhead. The three trails (Nalley, Brown, and Wetlands Trails) are all close to each other within the park, but the Nalley Trail is a 1.4-mile outer loop that gives you the best hiking experience.

Follow green trail markers into the park and begin the Nalley Trail to the right. The route is pretty flat and shady, with towering hardwoods, scrub pines, and other native plants. Vehicle noise from the nearby road is evident, but you'll still feel secluded within nature.

After making a small switchback, you'll see a fence that runs alongside a ravine and come to seven steps that lead across a wooden bridge to the left. Another bridge traverses the ravine. Soon, you'll have the option to go left onto the blue trail over the wetlands, but this hike continues forward with a slight uphill climb.

If you do choose to detour to the wetlands, just come back to this spot. The wetlands trail is alongside a tributary of Eighteen Mile Creek, which eventually makes its way to Lake Hartwell. Wildflowers, mosses, and ferns line the ravines and provide a cool, welcome respite in the summer.

As you reach the crest of the hill at 0.3 mile, a no-wire fence lines the trail as you catch glimpses of an adjacent meadow. Continue to another switchback. Keep to the right at the next break as you continue on the Nalley Trail.

You'll reach another fork here. Keep to the right as you continue to loop around. Depending on the season and day of the week, you may encounter families and others enjoying the trail or you may have it all to yourself.

This trail is perfect for families or those looking for an easy hike. If you want a longer outing, consider combining all three trails within the park, or hike this trail multiple times.

Nalley Brown Nature Park: Nalley Trail

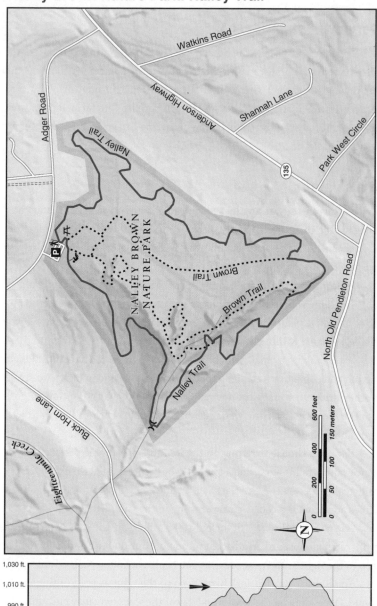

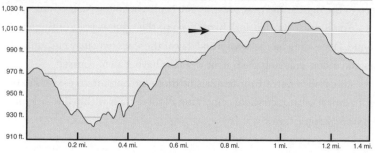

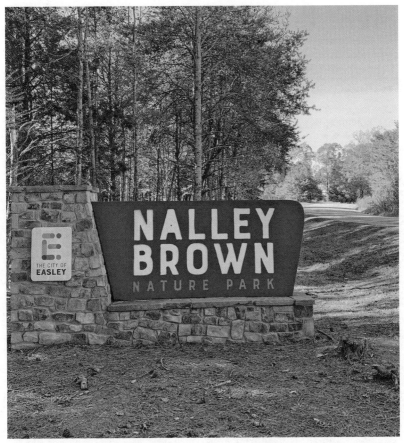

NALLEY BROWN NATURE PARK OFFERS EASY TRAILS THAT ARE GREAT FOR FAMILIES.

Nearby Attractions

Nalley Brown is near **Easley Silos,** a gathering spot with restaurants and a brewery built within decommissioned grain silos. Restaurants include **Inky's Authentic Cheesesteaks and Hoagies, Silos Brewery, Indigo Kitchen, Ninja Warrior Coffee House, Belladina's Pizzeria,** and **Pink Mama's Ice Cream.**

Directions

The trailhead is located at 380 Adger Road in Easley. From Greenville, take US 123 West approximately 18 miles to SC 135 South/South Pendleton Street in Easley. Continue on SC 135 South 1.9 miles to Adger Road and turn right. The entrance to the park is on your left.

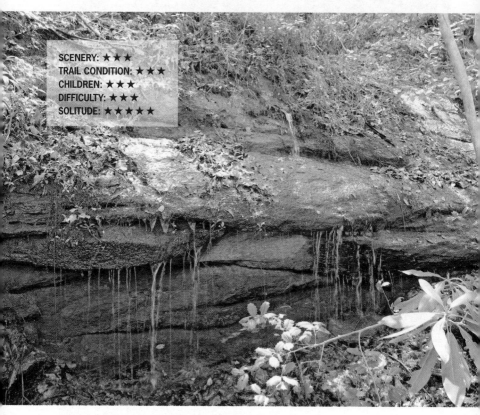

> SCENERY: ★ ★ ★
> TRAIL CONDITION: ★ ★ ★
> CHILDREN: ★ ★ ★
> DIFFICULTY: ★ ★ ★
> SOLITUDE: ★ ★ ★ ★ ★

A SMALL WATERFALL ALONG NINE TIMES PRESERVE TRAIL

TRAILHEAD GPS COORDINATES: N34° 56.913' W82° 47.539'

DISTANCE & CONFIGURATION: 4-mile out-and-back

HIKING TIME: 3 hours

HIGHLIGHTS: Seclusion, birder's paradise

ELEVATION: 1,169' at trailhead to 1,626' at peak, 0.7 mile into the hike at the top of the mountain

ACCESS: Daily, sunrise–sunset; free

MAPS: None

FACILITIES: None

WHEELCHAIR ACCESS: None

COMMENTS: The parking area is on the corner of Preston McDaniel Road and Nine Times Creek Road and is easy to miss, so keep an eye out.

CONTACT: The Nature Conservancy, nature.org

Overview

This is Pickens County's best trail for bird lovers. More than 110 species of birds have been logged in this 560-acre preserve since the trail opened in mid-2012. The area is also considered one of the most biologically significant areas in the southeast, with 134 species of native wildflowers, 130 different trees, and seven distinct forest types, and it is home to black bears, turkeys, and peregrine falcons. The trail follows old logging roads.

Route Details

Sometimes hiking is all about being out in nature alone, secluded, feeling like you're the only human in the world. Nine Times Preserve offers that feeling. It's definitely one of those "experience it now before other people find out about it" kind of places.

The 560 acres were part of a 2,300-acre parcel of land that Crescent Resources, a division of Duke Energy, had on the market. A coalition led by the Nature Conservancy realized the significance of the land and purchased the tract to preserve it for generations to come. The area is biologically significant due to its location, where the Piedmont landmass butts against the Blue Ridge Mountains, giving it a well-preserved diversity. Before the trail opened, the land had no trails and had limited public access known only to local hunters.

After you park in the small gravel parking area, go around the orange gates and follow the wide dirt path as it immediately begins uphill and to the right. You'll be following the Cedar Rock Trail here, which is fairly steep as you climb up the mountain, following an old logging road strewn with boulders and overgrown grasses. The road is still nearby, so the occasional passing car interrupts the solitude. Luckily, it's not a busy road.

Birds are plentiful, and aficionados can spend hours identifying the more than 110 species that have been documented here. Continue making your way up the steep mountainside. As you trek uphill, the trail becomes rockier. You can catch glimpses of the surrounding mountains through the trees. Little Pink Mountain, Rocky Bald Mountain, and Turkey Mountain are all visible.

Trail markers are few and far between, as there are only a few orange trail signs, but the path is still pretty easy to follow. When you get to the top of the mountain, stop and rest, as you've just climbed 400 feet.

At the top is a sign with the trail map. Turn right here to follow the Rocky Bald Loop Trail. As the trail narrows and levels out, you'll again notice how quiet

Nine Times Preserve

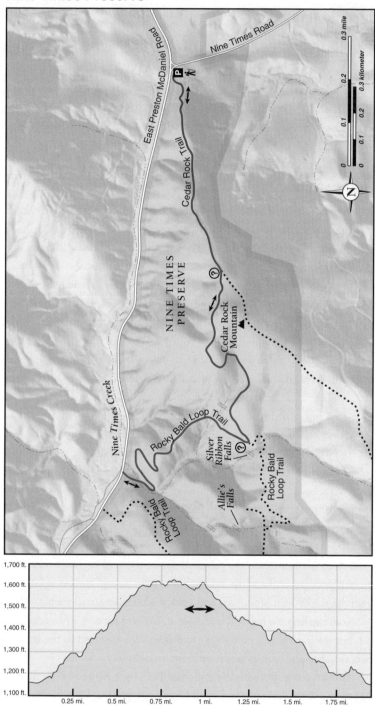

and secluded it is—the only sounds are the chirping of the birds in the trees. The trail follows along with the mountain to the left and a deep gorge on the right; on clear days you can see the Smoky Mountains in the distance.

Once you make it around the back side of the mountain, you begin downhill, with switchbacks making the descent easier than the beginning trail was. When you get to another trail sign, take the trail to the right. Soon you'll hear the water from nearby Nine Times Creek.

As you continue to descend on the switchbacks, 1.4 miles into the hike, you'll come to a small waterfall cascading over a rock with a small stream trickling down the mountain. Cross over and continue on the trail. Flowering rhododendrons are numerous, as are ferns and wildflowers. As you make your way closer to the bottom, you will once again hear traffic sounds and see the nearby roadway.

At the bottom of the trail, you come to Nine Times Creek as the pathway curves and takes you alongside the creek bank. Cross the creek on stones placed to aid your rock-hopping. Wooden stairs on the other side lead you up. When you get to the road and another parking area, turn around and head back.

Nearby Attractions

Nine Times Preserve is both a Nature Conservancy property and a South Carolina Wildlife Management Area, so hunting and fishing are allowed.

Directions

From Pickens, take US 178 north for 4.7 miles. Turn left onto Preston McDaniel Road and travel another 4.6 miles. The gravel parking area is at the corner of Preston McDaniel Road and Nine Times Creek Road.

Table Rock State Park: Carrick Creek Trail

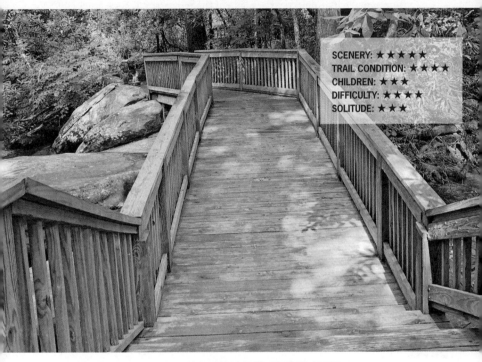

SCENERY: ★★★★★
TRAIL CONDITION: ★★★★
CHILDREN: ★★★
DIFFICULTY: ★★★★
SOLITUDE: ★★★

SEVERAL BRIDGES AND WALKWAYS CROSS OVER CARRICK CREEK.

TRAILHEAD GPS COORDINATES: N35° 01.917' W82° 42.047'

DISTANCE & CONFIGURATION: 2.2-mile balloon

HIKING TIME: 1.25 hours

HIGHLIGHTS: Several waterfalls and creeks

ELEVATION: 1,078' at the trailhead to 1,526' at peak

ACCESS: Sunday–Thursday, 7 a.m.–7 p.m.; Friday–Saturday, 7 a.m.–9 p.m. Daylight saving time: Sunday–Thursday, 7 a.m.–9 p.m.; Friday–Saturday, 7 a.m.–10 p.m.; $6 for age 16 and older; $3.75 for seniors; $3.50 for children ages 6–15; free for age 5 and younger

MAPS: Table Rock State Park, USGS *Table Rock State Park*

FACILITIES: Restrooms, water fountain, soda machine, and benches at the nature center

WHEELCHAIR ACCESS: None

COMMENTS: Dogs are allowed but must be on a 6-foot leash at all times. During summer the area gets busy and parking might be a little hard to find.

CONTACT: Table Rock State Park, 864-878-9813, southcarolinaparks.com/table-rock

Overview

This is my favorite area for hiking in all the Upstate. The location, just off SC 11, makes it easy to get to, and the views of Table Rock Mountain are spectacular. The trail follows along Carrick Creek for a good portion of the hike, and you'll pass several waterfalls and cross over the creek many times. While this trail is only a little over 2-miles, it is quite challenging, with some steep changes in elevation and several creek crossings. Even during the hot summer months, it is cooler here, and the shady path and water offer a welcome respite.

Route Details

All trails begin at the nature center. Be sure to register as a hiker before you begin. The area around the nature center can be busy, but once you get off the paved pathway and onto the trail, you may hike quite a while without seeing another person. The trip begins as a paved pathway, and you'll cross over Carrick Creek on the first of several bridges. The first waterfall you'll see is just a short walk, and a very popular swimming hole sits right beneath the falls. There are decks and benches here, and you'll find many families hanging out and enjoying the falls no matter the season. Head up the paved trail a short distance and you'll pass a second waterfall. Here there are a series of steps as you walk alongside the creek until you get to a second bridge. This is where you lose not only the paved pathway but also a majority of the people. Across the bridge is officially where the Carrick Creek Trail loop begins.

Follow the green markings to the left for Carrick Creek Trail as it shares a path with the Foothills Trail. Depending on the season, you may find gorgeous hydrangeas and bougainvillea blooming with white and pink flowers. The trail follows the creek for quite a while, crossing back and forth several times, and it's soothing to hear the water rushing across the rocks. Another set of natural steps leads you higher in elevation. Small streams trickle down the mountain in several areas, and it can be quite muddy if it has rained recently, so be sure to have appropriate shoes. The clay trail is also riddled with tree roots, so you will need to watch your footing at all times. After you've climbed for a short period, you'll come across a series of large smooth rocks. A wooden pathway winds around toward the sliding rock area. This area is popular with teenagers, and you can watch people sliding in the rushing water if the weather is warm. Continue on the series of wooden steps up and around to the left as you approach a 0.5-mile marker.

Table Rock State Park: Carrick Creek Trail

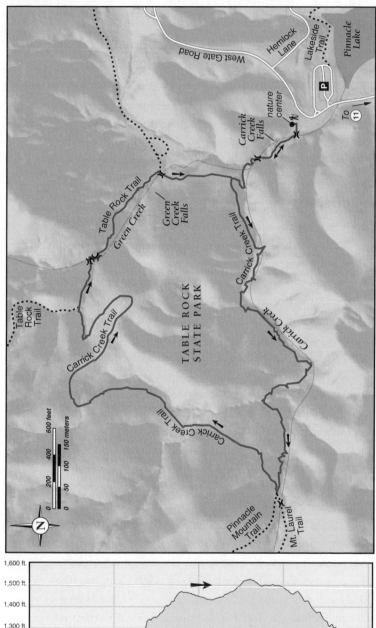

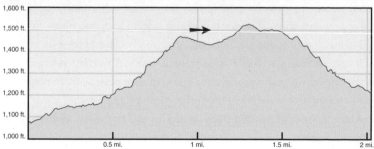

The trail starts to get pretty steep here as you continue to climb. The creek seems to disappear for a short time only to come out of the mountain at the next waterfall. After crossing another bridge you'll notice the light filtering through the trees more prominently as the elevation gets higher and you're closer to the sky. At this point you are still following the creek until you come to another fork. Here you can decide if you want to continue to the longer 4.1-mile Pinnacle Trail or the shorter Carrick Creek Trail Loop. For this hike take the Carrick Creek Trail Loop. The trail heads away from the water, and the pathway immediately gets wider as you slowly start descending. The sounds of water start to diminish as you begin to hear birds chirping and lizards scurrying in the underbrush. The hike becomes a little easier and you notice that you're actually on the back side of the mountain you just ascended. Pass over a very small stream as you start uphill again.

You're still at the top of the mountain, and you'll notice that the trees are younger and smaller up here. As you continue to descend you will hear the rushing water once more in the distance. The trail switchbacks as you continue your descent. There's another fork in the trail at 1.6 miles, where the Table Rock Trail goes to the left, but stay on the Carrick Creek Trail to the right. You'll come upon another bridge where you pick up Green Creek again and cross. Here's where you really start going downhill. Rocks serve as stairs and are fairly steep at times. The creek is to your right and yet another waterfall almost sneaks up on you. The path is narrower here, especially the steeper it gets, and blackberry bushes dot the trail. The trail continues down and starts to curve back around to the right. After another waterfall and bridge to cross it, you come back to where you began the loop portion of the hike. From here, retrace your route to the nature center.

Nearby Attractions

Table Rock State Park has five other trails you hike, including the **Table Rock Trail** (see next profile). **Pinnacle Lake** (right across the road from the trailheads) has kayak and canoe rentals during the summer. There are also cabins available for rent, and a swimming area with a diving board is open during the summer. **Aunt Sue's Country Corner,** about a mile east on SC 11, is a great place to stop for a bite to eat or enjoy some ice cream while you're in the area.

Directions

From Greenville take US 276 to SC 11 and go west about 6.6 miles. There is a visitor center on the left, but the trailheads are all to the right. You will see a sign that says TABLE ROCK STATE PARK WEST ENTRANCE.

From I-26, take SC Exit 5 onto SC 11 toward Campobello. All trailheads begin at the nature center, and a large parking area is directly across the road.

TABLE ROCK MOUNTAIN

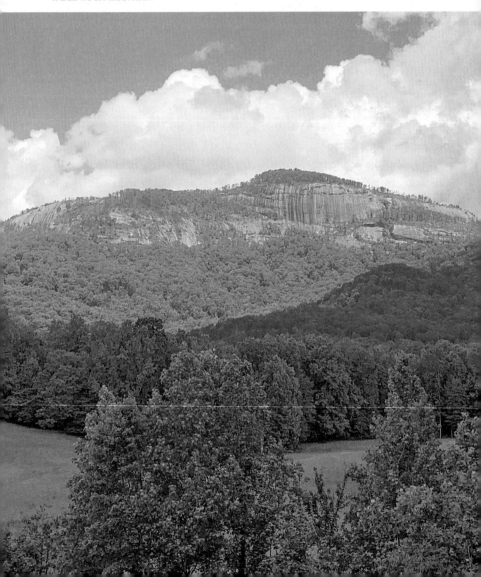

12 # Table Rock State Park:
Table Rock Trail

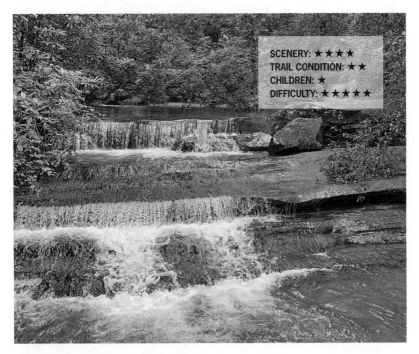

> SCENERY: ★★★★
> TRAIL CONDITION: ★★
> CHILDREN: ★
> DIFFICULTY: ★★★★

WATERFALLS AT TABLE ROCK STATE PARK

TRAILHEAD GPS COORDINATES: N35° 01.924' W82° 42.018'

DISTANCE & CONFIGURATION: 8.6-mile out-and-back

HIKING TIME: 7.25 hours

HIGHLIGHTS: Mountain views, challenging hike

ELEVATION: 1,145' at trailhead to 3,124' at the summit sign

ACCESS: Sunday–Thursday, 7 a.m.–7 p.m.; Friday–Saturday, 7 a.m.–9 p.m. Daylight saving time: Sunday–Thursday, 7 a.m.–9 p.m.; Friday–Saturday, 7 a.m.–10 p.m.; $6 for age 16 and older; $3.75 for seniors; $3.50 for children ages 6–15; free for age 5 and younger

MAPS: Table Rock State Park, USGS *Table Rock State Park*

FACILITIES: Restrooms, water fountain, soda machine, and benches at the nature center

WHEELCHAIR ACCESS: None

COMMENTS: Dogs are allowed but must be on a 6-foot leash at all times. During summer months the area gets busy and parking might be a little hard to find. Ranger programs throughout the year offer sunrise and moonlight hikes.

CONTACT: Table Rock State Park, 864-878-9813, southcarolinaparks.com/table-rock

Table Rock State Park: Table Rock Trail

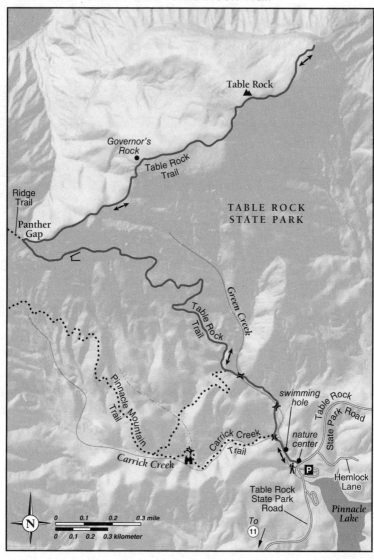

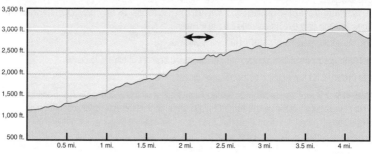

Overview

This trail should be on the bucket list of every hiker who lives or visits the Upstate. There are definite bragging rights to be claimed as you climb over boulders, navigate tree roots, climb the face of Governor's Rock, and make your way 2,000 feet to the summit of Table Rock. Even the most serious hiker will find the hike challenging and rewarding. Once atop the large granite rock, hikers are compensated with amazing views of the surrounding mountains, a nearby watershed, and, on clear days, the City of Greenville.

Route Details

Legend has it that Table Rock was named *Sah-ka-na-ga* by a giant Cherokee chieftain who, when finished hunting, would stop here and use the Table Rock Mountain as his dining table while sitting on nearby Stool Mountain to eat his venison. Today, this lush and green forest, with its many streams and boulders, is a popular playground for the Upstate with its 3,000 acres and many facilities. Many of Table Rock's cabins and structures built by the Civilian Conservation Corps (CCC) are on the National Register of Historic Places.

Begin the hike at the nature center (be sure to register as a hiker) and follow alongside Carrick Creek, passing multiple waterfalls, until you get to a fork. Table Rock serves as an access point to the 80-mile Foothills Trail, and if you take the trail to the left, you can access the Foothills Trail and the Carrick Creek Trail. Table Rock Trail is the only trail that goes to the right. Continue to the right as the dirt trail ascends gradually and then heads slightly downhill.

The trail has some tree roots encroaching on the path and wooden reinforcements but is generally in good condition. As you continue, Green Creek will be on the right. You'll soon come to a wooden footbridge that crosses the creek, and on the other side are stone rocks that serve as a staircase as you begin to travel uphill. As the trail curves around, the creek is now on the left. Continue uphill with stones as steps to assist. The trail is well marked with both green and red markers. The green is for Carrick Creek Trail, as this is the end of the loop portion of that trail, but you want to follow the red trail markers.

After you pass several more waterfalls, another wooden footbridge will take you across Green Creek. As the trail continues its uphill climb, you'll reach the 0.5-mile trail sign and swear that you've already hiked several miles as you continue upward. Just past that sign you'll come to another fork. This is where

Carrick Creek Trail veers to the left. Continue to the right as you leave the creek, following the TABLE ROCK sign and red trail markers.

Pass over a couple of small streams as you continue your journey up. If it has rained recently, the trail can be muddy here, so watch your footing carefully. As you continue to wind and climb, you'll pass by several large boulders. It's quiet with only the wind in the trees and birds singing. At 1 mile you reach a small summit as the path levels out a little. Enjoy glimpses of the surrounding mountains through the trees, and even on busy days with nice weather there is still a feeling of solitude.

The trail continues winding around on a mostly uphill trek with just a few feet of leveling out. You will have gone up so many stone steps that you'll have lost count by now. Large boulders continue to dot the landscape as you climb over and walk past several boulders nestled among the trees as you continue up and up. When you get to the CCC shelter, you're at about the halfway point, at 2.3 miles. Wooden benches provide seating, and there's a nice overlook with views of the surrounding mountains and valley below.

Continue uphill until you get to Panther Gap. This is where the Ridge Trail (with orange blazes) and Table Rock Trail meet up. Continue to the right, following the red blazes. Here the trail levels out as you begin to walk along the ridge of the mountain. The path is mostly level with a few ups and downs. At 2.5 miles the trail heads uphill again. After a steep, rocky climb you'll be atop Governor's Rock, a massive flat rock atop Table Rock. It can be a little tricky to maneuver, but luckily there are small carved indentations to assist. Once you scale the massive rock, the trail levels out as you are pretty near the top.

After another steep climb, you arrive at the summit. You will know this because there is a large sign. Make sure to get a photo to prove that you indeed conquered Table Rock and made it to the top. This is the highest point on the mountain, but you're not quite done with the hike. Go about a quarter mile more downhill and you'll come to a massive flat rock area with spectacular views overlooking a watershed. On clear days you can see Paris Mountain and downtown Greenville, and you'll look around and say, "Yeah, that was worth it."

There's no way around it, you have to go back down the 2,000 feet you just climbed. At least going down is faster for most people, and if you're anything like me, sunlight will be starting to fade, which will push you to hike even faster.

Nearby Attractions

Table Rock State Park has five other trails you hike, including the **Carrick Creek Trail** (see previous profile). **Pinnacle Lake** (right across the road from the trailheads) has kayak and canoe rentals during the summer. There are also cabins available for rent, and a swimming area with a diving board is open during the summer. **Aunt Sue's Country Corner,** about a mile east on SC 11, is a great place to stop for a bite to eat or enjoy some ice cream while you're in the area.

Directions

From Greenville take US 276 to SC 11 and go west about 6.6 miles. A visitor center is on the left, but the trailheads are all to the right. You will see a sign that says TABLE ROCK STATE PARK WEST ENTRANCE.

From I-26, take SC Exit 5 onto SC 11 toward Campobello. All trailheads begin at the nature center, and a large parking area is directly across the road.

SIGNAGE ALONG THE TABLE ROCK TRAIL

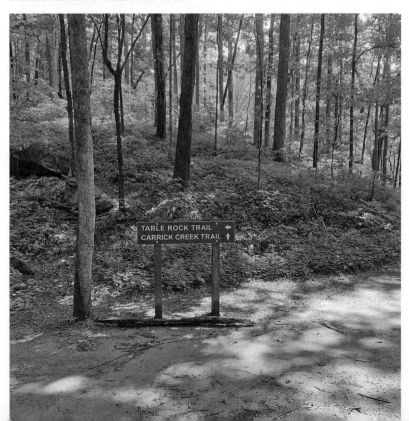

Greenville County (Hikes 13–21)

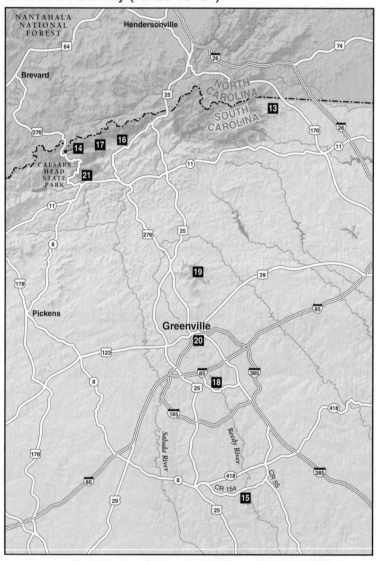

Greenville County

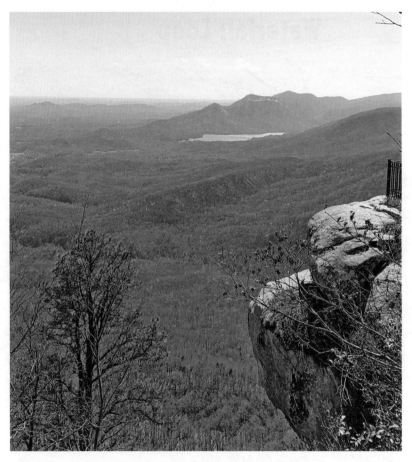

VIEW FROM CAESARS HEAD OVERLOOK *(See Hike 14, page 82.)*

Blue Wall Passage of the Palmetto Trail and Waterfall Loop

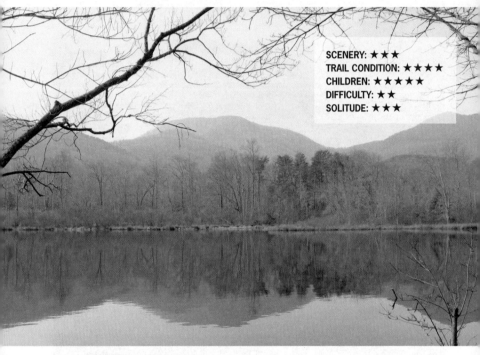

SCENERY: ★★★
TRAIL CONDITION: ★★★★
CHILDREN: ★★★★★
DIFFICULTY: ★★
SOLITUDE: ★★★

TWIN PONDS ALONG THE BLUE WALL PASSAGE

TRAILHEAD GPS COORDINATES: N35° 11.072' W82° 14.897'

DISTANCE & CONFIGURATION: 3.2-mile balloon

HIKING TIME: 2.25 hours

HIGHLIGHTS: Mountain views, lake views, waterfall

ELEVATION: 1,155' at trailhead to 1,396' at waterfall

ACCESS: Daily, sunrise–sunset; free

MAPS: palmettoconservation.org, palmettotrail.org

FACILITIES: None

WHEELCHAIR ACCESS: None

COMMENTS: Dogs are allowed. No mountain biking, camping, or fires permitted.

CONTACT: Palmetto Conservation Foundation, 803-771-0870, palmettoconservation.org/passage/blue-wall-passage

Overview

Blue Wall Passage is part of the Palmetto Trail, a 500-mile project that, when completed, will be South Carolina's largest bicycle and pedestrian trail system. The Palmetto Trail features primitive pathways along mountaintops, forests, and some rail-to-trail conversions. The Blue Wall Passage, named for its drastic and sudden 3,000-foot shift in elevation, forming an abrupt "blue wall," is at the easternmost portion of the Blue Ridge Escarpment and provides captivating views of the surrounding mountains, lakes, and a waterfall.

Route Details

From the parking area, walk past the gate and down the paved roadway about 0.2 mile. The roadway will end as you come to a trailhead sign after crossing over a small creek. The inviting sound of rushing water and the sight of the surrounding mountains will put you in the mood for a great outing.

The Blue Wall Preserve sign is large and dominating and an indication to proceed straight onto the dirt path. You'll cross another gate over another creek before you come to the actual trailhead sign. Continue straight on the gravel and dirt roadway as you begin a slight uphill climb.

You'll continue along the old road, which is now only open to foot traffic. There is a gully to the left, a hillside to your right, and you can still hear the gurgling of the stream. Soon you come to another gate and a fork. Roads lead to the right and straight ahead here. Follow the old road straight ahead, marked with a palmetto sign and yellow trail markers on the trees.

Soon you arrive at a small lake marked with an interpretive sign. Enjoy the great views of Hogback Mountain here. Hogback Mountain is part of South Carolina's Dark Corner, made famous by its illegal moonshiners. Rumor has it that there are still moonshine stills hidden deep in the mountain.

There is another fork here with a trail to the left that will take you along the lake for a short distance, but you should continue forward on the path. The road is more overgrown here as it becomes a wide pathway instead of road. As you continue around the lake, the trail is mostly level. Trees on both sides become more abundant as you once again hear the rushing creek to the left, although you can't see it, and the chirping of birds overhead becomes louder as you immerse yourself in the natural surroundings.

When you come to the first of two ponds, called Twin Ponds, you'll be at another fork on the pathway, approximately 1.2 miles into the hike. This is the

Blue Wall Passage of the Palmetto Trail & Waterfall Loop

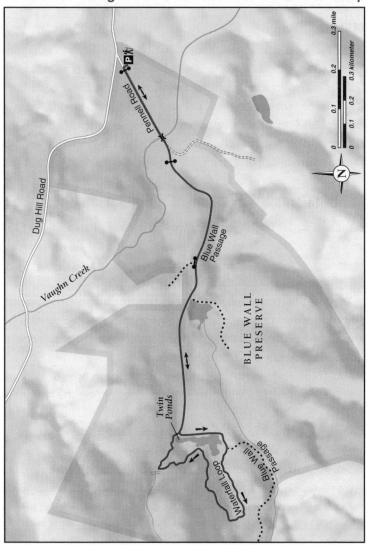

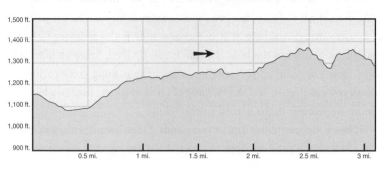

loop portion of the trail, so you can go either way. We took the path to the left (south). The trail will wind around the water, and when you get about halfway around there will be yet another fork. Here you could continue straight and take a much longer and strenuous hike up through Vaughns Gap, but this hike continues to the right around the two ponds.

The trail is narrower here as it continues to wind around with the pond to your right. The path is mostly level but is littered with tree roots. As you make your way around the loop, follow the metal signs to the right as the trail begins to descend. It can be muddy here, especially if it has rained recently.

The path begins a slight ascent, and as you round the corner, the trail becomes wider and the trees sparser before you travel slightly downhill again. The mountains are to your right now. You'll return to the pond, but this time on the other side. The trail continues around, skirting the edge of the pond as it gradually turns into a small creek as you observe several beaver dams.

The small waterfall soon appears on your left, cascading about 25 feet over several rocks. This is a good place to stop to rest and take photos before you continue over the small concrete slab footbridge to your right. Just past the waterfall you will close the loop portion of the trail. Continue back on the trail that you came in on.

Nearby Attractions

For a much longer and more strenuous hike (with 1,500 feet of elevation gain within 3 miles), continue on the Palmetto Trail for another 11 miles, going up through **Vaughns Gap** and connecting to the **Poinsett Reservoir Passage.**

Directions

Take I-26 North to Exit 1 (right before the North Carolina state line). Turn left (west) onto SC 14 toward Landrum. Turn right onto US 176 for about 2 miles. Turn left onto West Lakeshore Drive and drive around the lake. The parking area and trailhead will be on your right on Dug Hill Road.

14 # Caesars Head State Park: Raven Cliff Falls

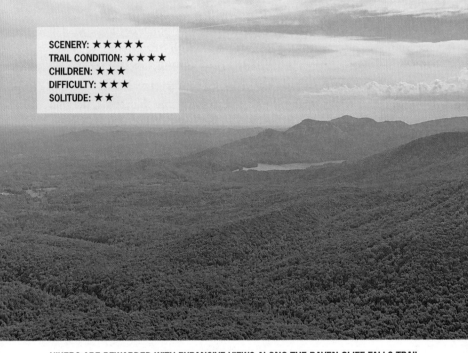

SCENERY: ★★★★★
TRAIL CONDITION: ★★★★
CHILDREN: ★★★
DIFFICULTY: ★★★
SOLITUDE: ★★

HIKERS ARE REWARDED WITH EXPANSIVE VIEWS ALONG THE RAVEN CLIFF FALLS TRAIL.

TRAILHEAD GPS COORDINATES: N35° 06.943' W82° 38.291'

DISTANCE & CONFIGURATION: 4.4-mile out-and-back

HIKING TIME: 3.25 hours

HIGHLIGHTS: Magnificent views, creeks, and a waterfall

ELEVATION: 2,866' at trailhead to 3,165' about 1 mile into the hike

ACCESS: Daily, Raven Cliff Falls parking area 9 a.m.–6 p.m. Daylight saving time: daily, 9 a.m.–9 p.m. Trails close one hour before dark, year-round. $3 for age 16 and older; $1.50 for SC seniors; $1 for children ages 6–15; free for age 5 and younger

MAPS: USGS *Table Rock State Park,* South Carolina Parks, Mountain Bridge Wilderness Area

FACILITIES: Restrooms at the Caesars Head visitor center

WHEELCHAIR ACCESS: None

COMMENTS: Dogs are allowed but must be leashed. On weekends the parking lot can fill quickly. There are no trash cans, so please pack out what you bring.

CONTACT: Caesars Head State Park, 864-836-6115, southcarolinaparks.com/caesars-head

Overview

Caesars Head is one of South Carolina's most famous natural landmarks, with sweeping views of the surrounding mountains. The Raven Cliff Falls Trail is part of the 10,000-acre Mountain Bridge Wilderness trail system and Foothills Trail and is one of the most popular hikes at Caesars Head. The moderately difficult trail leads to an overlook where you can view the 420-foot Raven Cliff Falls in the distance.

Route Details

A granite gneiss (a major metamorphic rock) outcrop atop the dramatic Blue Ridge Escarpment gives Caesars Head State Park its name. It's worth stopping at the visitor center to not only pay the hiking fee but also take in the amazing views from the overlook areas. If visiting during Hawk Watch (September 1–November 30), you can watch migrating raptors soar above the trees. If the visitor center is not open, envelopes are available at the parking area to pay the hiking fee on an honor system.

You can either park at the visitor center or at the Raven Cliff Falls parking area. If parking in the Raven Cliff Falls parking area, you must cross US 276 to get to the trailhead. The trailhead begins at the highway. The first section of trail follows an old carriage road, so it is quite wide and graded. Several other trails also begin from this location, so make sure you are following the red trail blazes.

You immediately begin to descend, and the air suddenly seems cooler as the trail takes you through a forest of ferns. At the Caesars Head Water Company Building the trail veers to the right. Here the path becomes narrower, and you can hear rushing water from the small creek that you will be passing over. Tree roots begin to encroach on the dirt trail as it starts to wind around and begin an uphill approach following the edge of the mountain.

As you make your way alongside the mountain, don't miss the magnificent views through the trees. As you start a gradual descent, you will lose the sound of the highway and begin to hear the rushing of the falls in the distance. At about 0.6 mile turn right, away from the mountain edge you have been following. Since you have been climbing in elevation, you will begin to notice more pine trees.

As you make your way across some rocks (don't worry—they are mostly flat and easy to walk on) you will come to a set of stairs at 0.8 mile. The trail turns back toward the left as the descent gets steeper; the tree canopy is higher

Caesars Head State Park: Raven Cliff Falls

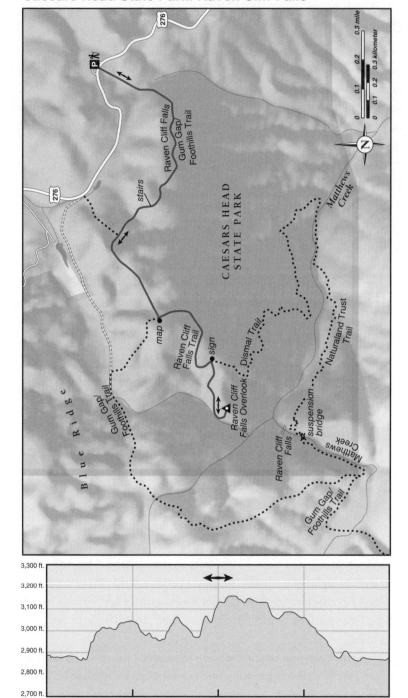

and less light filters in. You encounter a lot of ups and downs in the path as you walk along a small creek deep in the forest. Soon, though, you'll be at the top of the mountain again and start to weave around it. The trail becomes sandy here and evens out for a little while. At a crossroads where the blue trail goes right and the red trail (Raven Cliff Falls) goes left, stay on the red trail.

As the path levels out a little more, you'll come to a sign identifying the trail. Unless you are feeling very adventurous, do not go to the left, which is the purple Dismal Trail. That trail is very strenuous and will add another four hours to your hike. Continue on the red trail to the right and soon you will reach a nice overlook with benches and Raven Cliff Falls in the background. It's important to note that you do not get up close to this waterfall; it's quite a way off in the distance, and depending on rainfall, the waterfall may not be as spectacular as others in the area. Once you've rested, turn around and return the way you came. As you return, you may notice cairns, or "hiker art." These are collections of rocks stacked upon each other. Be sure to stop and add your own contribution.

Nearby Attractions

While at Caesars Head, be sure to visit the overlooks for amazing views. There are also picnic tables and several other hikes varying in length that leave from this area. Check in with the rangers at the visitor center for a detailed trail map and information.

Caesars Head connects to **Jones Gap State Park** (see hikes on pages 90–97) in what is known as the **Mountain Bridge Wilderness Area,** an 11,000-acre area of pristine southern mountain forest. Hikers can take a number of trails that connect the parks, and trailside camping is available for those who choose the longer routes.

Directions

From Greenville take US 276 west for approximately 32 miles. Follow the signs toward Caesars Head. The parking area for Raven Cliff Falls is on the right side of US 276 just past the Caesars Head Visitor Center.

Cedar Falls Park Trail

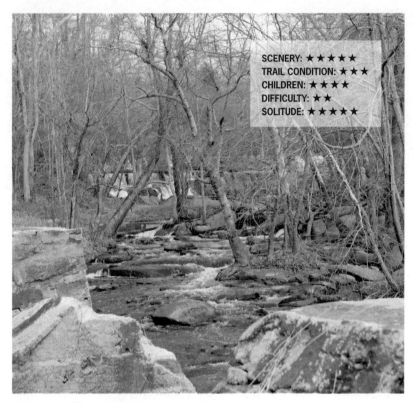

CEDAR FALLS AND THE REEDY RIVER

SCENERY: ★★★★★
TRAIL CONDITION: ★★★
CHILDREN: ★★★★
DIFFICULTY: ★★
SOLITUDE: ★★★★★

TRAILHEAD GPS COORDINATES: N34° 36.734' W82° 17.925'

DISTANCE & CONFIGURATION: 1.9-mile balloon

HIKING TIME: 1.5 hours

HIGHLIGHTS: Historic site, cascading waterfalls, Reedy River

ELEVATION: 642' at trailhead to 740' at top of hill

ACCESS: Daily, 9 a.m.–sunset or 7 p.m.; free

MAPS: Greenville Recreation

FACILITIES: Restrooms, picnic facilities, and playground at the park area

WHEELCHAIR ACCESS: Not on the trail

COMMENTS: Dogs are allowed but must be leashed. The trail is also open to equestrians. Signs are posted indicating that swimming is discouraged, but many ignore them. Be sure to wear insect repellent during warmer months.

CONTACT: Greenville County Recreation District, greenvillerec.com/parks/cedar-falls

Overview

The shoals at Cedar Falls were used to power local mills and in the 1820s to generate electrical power. Today it's a Greenville County park with cascading waterfalls dumping into numerous pools. Few locals even knew the falls existed, but that changed in 2011 when the park received a $2.7 million makeover thanks to funds left over from the cleanup of a 1996 oil spill, the largest ever in South Carolina, which dumped more than a million gallons of diesel fuel into the Reedy River. Cedar Falls Park is maintained by the Greenville County Recreation District and includes picnic shelters, restrooms, a playground, and a sand volleyball court.

Route Details

This Greenville County park is still relatively unknown except to nearby residents. There are two sections, the main park area and the falls area. Begin by driving past Cedar Falls Park and park in the small lot at the waterfall.

As soon as you get out of the car, you will be amazed by the expansive cascades of the falls. Reminiscent of a small Niagara Falls, the Reedy River widens to more than 200 feet here with water cascading over numerous rocks and boulders. The site itself is historic. In the 1800s, Native Americans used the rock shoals as a hunting campsite and as a way to cross the river. Also in the 1800s, Hudson Berry built a dam to feed a waterwheel that powered his textile mill, grist mill, sawmill, and cotton gin. The stone foundations of these still exist today.

In 1910 a bigger dam and power plant were built across the entire river to produce electrical power for the Fork Shoals Mill, a home, and a medical clinic. The mills were operational until the 1940s, when Fork Shoals Mill began buying electrical power from Duke Power, and in 1950 the power plant was demolished.

After you are finished looking around the falls, take the trail to the left. Notice the four interpretive signs on your right that tell of the history and natural environment of the falls. The wide, paved pathway starts off slightly uphill as you soon come to a nice view overlooking the falls at the dam. There is a bench here if you need to rest or just reflect on the natural beauty surrounding you.

Keep following the path and soon you come to a fork. This will eventually tie Cedar Falls Park and Cedar Falls together. Continue straight ahead until the pavement ends and you come upon another bench. This bench overlooks the Reedy River.

Follow the trail to the left as it turns to dirt but is still fairly wide. The ground is level here as you walk through the forest, leaving the falls behind.

Cedar Falls Park Trail

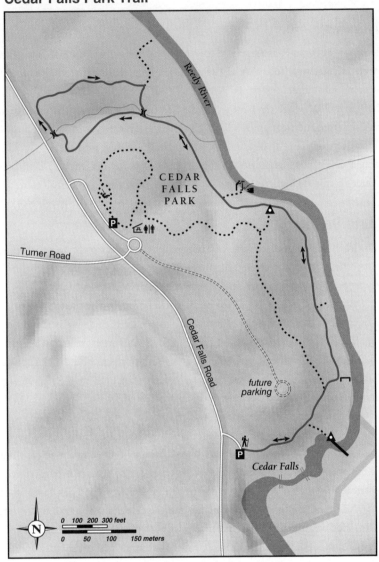

Soon you come to another fork; continue to the right as you follow along the river. It's quiet and still here, except for the birds calling to each other as they fly through the treetops and bushes.

Soon you come to yet another fork where the path either goes up the hill to the left or down to the river to the right. Take the path up the hill to the left. As you continue slightly uphill the trail evens out as you begin walking along the rim with the river now below.

As you begin to head slightly downhill, the river will be on your right, but you won't be able to see it. At the next fork continue to the right until you come to yet another fork. This time go left. You'll begin to hear sounds of the nearby road and know that you have once again entered civilization.

At the next fork, if you go left, it will take you up to the far-left section of Cedar Falls Park. Continue on the path to the right. You'll soon come to a small bridge over a stream as you walk right alongside the road to the left. This doesn't last long, as the trail will turn right, away from the road. The path here is wide, and it's evident that park vehicles use this section.

At 0.7 mile the trail goes uphill slightly before descending as you begin to loop around and head back. You'll come to another fork. To the left is what looks like an old tree fort, so continue to the right. The trail heads slightly to the right as you cross a bridge back over the small creek that you crossed earlier as you complete the loop. From here, continue along the same pathway you came in on to return to your car.

Nearby Attractions

Cedar Falls Park has a playground, a sand volleyball court, and picnic shelters.

Directions

The park is located at 201 Cedar Falls Road in Fountain Inn. From Greenville, take I-385 to Fairview Road to SC 418 and turn right. Turn left on Fork Shoals Road and then make another left on McKelvey Road. Take a right onto Cedar Falls Road and look for the park on the left. Cedar Falls is about 24 miles from downtown Greenville.

16 # Jones Gap State Park: Falls Trail

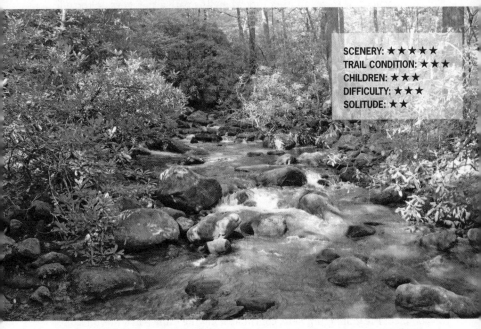

SCENERY: ★★★★★
TRAIL CONDITION: ★★★
CHILDREN: ★★★
DIFFICULTY: ★★★
SOLITUDE: ★★

A TRIBUTARY OF THE MIDDLE SALUDA RIVER FLOWS THROUGH JONES GAP STATE PARK.

TRAILHEAD GPS COORDINATES: N35° 07.532' W82° 34.302"

DISTANCE & CONFIGURATION: 3.2-mile out-and-back

HIKING TIME: 2.75 hours

HIGHLIGHTS: Great scenery along the Middle Saluda River, waterfall

ELEVATION: 2,145' at trailhead, with no significant elevation change

ACCESS: Daily, 9 a.m.–6 p.m. Daylight saving time: daily, 9 a.m.–9 p.m.; December 1–September 30: $6 for age 16 and older; $3.75 for SC seniors; $3.50 for ages 6–15; free for age 5 and younger

MAPS: South Carolina State Park Mountain Bridge Wilderness Area

FACILITIES: Restrooms and picnic benches at the Jones Gap State Park Visitor Center, which is open 9 a.m.–4 p.m. daily

WHEELCHAIR ACCESS: None

COMMENTS: For a memorable hiking experience, combine this route with the Jones Gap State Park: Rainbow Falls Trail (p. 94). Cell phone service is very spotty in the area. Parking can be limited in peak season and may require a reservation. Please check the SC State Park website for details.

CONTACT: Jones Gap State Park, 864-836-3647, southcarolinaparks.com/jones-gap

Overview

With more than 60 miles of trails, Jones Gap State Park offers a lot of choices. This hike covers a pleasant, moderately strenuous route that traverses boulders, passes several streams, and follows alongside the Saluda River. A toll road built in the 1840s and in use until 1910, the path follows the Middle Saluda River downstream. Now riddled with boulders, the trail looks more like an old creekbed than a road—and thus makes for an interesting journey.

Route Details

The entire Jones Gap National Recreation Trail is more than 5 miles one way and connects to Caesars Head State Park (page 82). This 3.2-mile route follows the Jones Gap National Recreation Trail to a spur for the Jones Gap waterfall and then returns to the visitor center. It also provides a different experience from the Jones Gap State Park: Rainbow Falls Trail hike (page 94).

Begin at the trailhead just past the visitor center. All trails are well marked, and you will follow the *blue* blazes to begin. (To avoid confusion, note that you will follow the *red* blazes for the Jones Gap State Park: Rainbow Falls Trail.) The pathway is a little sandy at the beginning as it follows along a rocky creek. Soon you encounter several large boulders to maneuver over as you pass some walk-in campsites along the Middle Saluda River. This river was South Carolina's first designated Scenic River and is a popular fishing hole, with a large population of trout. Also, a portion of Jones Gap is located on the Eastern Continental Divide, which means that water from part of the river will eventually flow into the Atlantic Ocean, while other portions will end up in the Gulf of Mexico.

Continue along the trail for a while as you follow the river on your right. It's hard to believe that this was ever a roadway. It has been rumored that Solomon Jones, who was a self-taught mountain road builder, used a hatchet and followed the lead of a pig to build the road. The unpaved road was abandoned by 1910 in favor of Geer Highway and now looks more like an old creekbed than a once-bustling toll road.

There are numerous tent-camping sites along the river. Camping is popular at Jones Gap, with travelers hiking the 77-mile-long Foothills Trail often using this area as a resting point. After crossing over a small creek, you encounter a fork in the trail. Continue following the blue blazes for Jones Gap Trail. The trail curves left, away from the river, and starts uphill. After coming to a crest,

Jones Gap State Park: Falls Trail

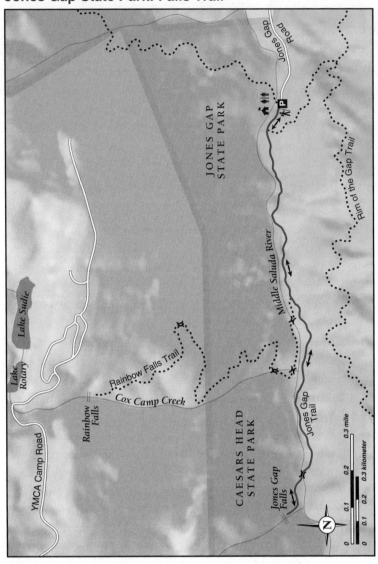

you'll walk along the creek as you descend again. Once you cross another creek, the trail levels off and becomes fairly wide for a short distance.

When you begin to climb again, the trail narrows and you notice how much higher in elevation you are. You can still hear the rushing water from the creeks, but water won't be visible until you turn the corner and see a bridge over the river. Once across the river you'll see another primitive campsite. Head to the left following the path and go another 200 yards. Cross the creek again and turn toward the left again following the sign to Jones Gap Falls.

The path becomes fairly steep, but luckily, it's only a short distance to the waterfall. Cross a small, flat wooden bridge over a consistently muddy section of the trail. A final short stretch brings you to the base of the 40-foot waterfall. The water cascades over several large, flat rocks that funnel the rushing water into a steady stream. Many flat boulders provide nice spots to sit and watch the waterfall cascade down the rocky cliff into the pool below. On a warm day, the shallow pool beneath the falls is a perfect place to cool off. When you're ready, hike back the same way you came in. You'll pass the trail signs for Rainbow Falls—consider doing both hikes while you are in the area.

Nearby Attractions

The **Cleveland Fish Hatchery** is located at Jones Gap State Park. Signs around the trout pond provide information on the 60–80 different types of trout that are on exhibit.

Directions

From Greenville, take US 276 north toward North Carolina. About 2 miles north of Cleveland, turn right at the Jones Gap sign onto River Falls Road. Follow River Falls Road for about 6 miles as it winds around and changes to Jones Gap Road. From the parking lot, follow the short trail to the Jones Gap Visitor Center.

17 Jones Gap State Park: Rainbow Falls Trail

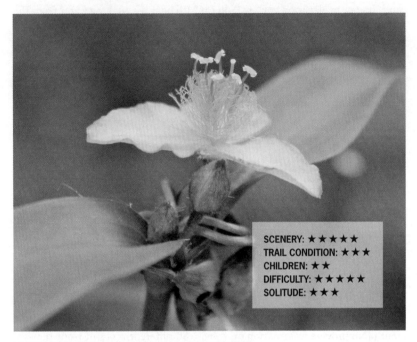

SCENERY: ★ ★ ★ ★ ★
TRAIL CONDITION: ★ ★ ★
CHILDREN: ★ ★
DIFFICULTY: ★ ★ ★ ★ ★
SOLITUDE: ★ ★ ★

LOOK FOR WILDFLOWERS ALONG RAINBOW FALLS TRAIL.

TRAILHEAD GPS COORDINATES: N35° 07.532' W82° 34.302'

DISTANCE & CONFIGURATION: 5-mile out-and-back

HIKING TIME: 5 hours

HIGHLIGHTS: Spectacular waterfall, challenging hike

ELEVATION: 2,145' at trailhead to 2,528' on ridge crest at the waterfall

ACCESS: Daily, 9 a.m.–6 p.m. Daylight saving time: daily, 9 a.m.–9 p.m.; December 1–September 30: $6 for age 16 and older; $3.75 for SC seniors; $3.50 for ages 6–15; free for age 5 and younger

MAPS: South Carolina State Park Mountain Bridge Wilderness Area

FACILITIES: Restrooms and picnic benches are available at the Jones Gap State Park Visitor Center, which is open 9 a.m.–4 p.m. daily.

WHEELCHAIR ACCESS: None

COMMENTS: Dogs are allowed but must be leashed. For a memorable hiking experience, combine this route with the Jones Gap State Park: Falls Trail (p. 90). Parking can be limited in peak season and may require a reservation. Please check the SC State Park website for details. Cell phone service is very spotty in the area.

CONTACT: Jones Gap State Park, 864-836-3647, southcarolinaparks.com/jones-gap

Overview

Part of the 11,000-acre Mountain Bridge Wilderness Area, Jones Gap State Park is a peaceful yet popular area with its five waterfalls and numerous trails. Rainbow Falls has been a favorite hiking destination for years, especially with campers from the nearby YMCA Camp Greenville. There's even an alternate route to the falls accessed through the campgrounds. Don't let the short distance on this hike fool you. It's a very steep elevation change, and you will be crawling over boulders. But it's definitely worth it—the waterfall is the best in South Carolina.

Route Details

The trailhead begins just to the left of the visitor center. Start here and follow the *red-blazed* trail. (To avoid confusion, note that you will follow the *blue* blazes for the Jones Gap State Park: Falls Trail hike, page 90.) The trail starts off fairly flat, wide, and sandy, heading west, but that doesn't last for long as you cross over a small stream and then a bridge over the Middle Saluda River. Here you follow along with the creek on your left. The trail remains quite level as you traverse the old toll road with many small boulders to navigate along the way.

Soon you'll come upon a one-log bridge that crosses over the river. The trail turns to the right after you cross the bridge, and there will be another smaller stream now as you cross over yet another footbridge, approximately 1.2 miles into the hike.

The trail leads to a huge boulder that you need to maneuver around. Don't worry, though, the trail winds around and gets a little tight in spots but it's passable. If you're really adventurous you can try to climb up and over the boulder, as I saw several kids do. On the other side of the boulder, you will turn toward the right and go up a fairly steep natural staircase. Continue following the red trail blazes as the route switches back and forth a few times. There will be two more sets of stairs as you continue your ascent.

The trail continues north, steeply climbing and switchbacking. The sound of rushing water from the creeks and streams becomes distant as you climb above the treetops. Rhododendron and mountain laurel canopy the landscape. In fall, this is also a popular place to view songbirds and raptors during their migratory trek. Ravens, falcons, and bald eagles are commonly spotted as well. The trail is overgrown at times and doesn't seem like a trail at all as you climb over rocks and boulders along the ridgeline of the mountain.

Jones Gap State Park: Rainbow Falls Trail

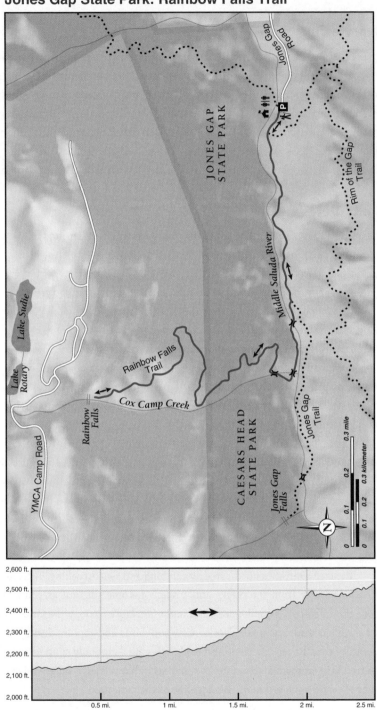

Pass a large rock face while you are still climbing and cross another small stream to ascend another series of stairs. Once you reach the top of these stairs, the trail widens a bit, and while you are still going uphill, it's not quite as steep as what you just accomplished.

You'll begin to hear the rushing of the waterfall before you see it, and as you round the last corner, the falls will come into view. The roar of the falls becomes almost deafening as you approach, and the temperature immediately drops from the mist, even on a hot summer day. If visiting during the winter months, be careful of icy patches. As the rushing water from Cox Camp Creek plunges over the granite walls, you will view the amazing 140-foot waterfall cascading down the mountain. This is by far the best waterfall hike in South Carolina. The feeling of accomplishment from tackling a challenging hike combined with the spectacular falls creates an incredible experience. Several rocks at the base of the falls provide a nice spot to sit and rest or have a picnic. There are even areas where you can climb right up next to and beneath the waterfall, but be careful, as these areas can get pretty slick.

This is an out-and-back, so when you're ready, return the way you came. The return trip is much easier, as a good majority of it is now downhill.

Nearby Attractions

Jones Gap State Park has more than 60 miles of trails, so you can enjoy other hikes or maybe a picnic near the **Cleveland Fish Hatchery.** This hike is also close to **Caesars Head State Park** (page 82), where you can take a nice drive to one of the overlook areas for sweeping, panoramic views of the South Carolina mountains, Georgia, and North Carolina.

Directions

From Greenville, take US 276 north toward North Carolina. About 2 miles north of Cleveland, turn right at the Jones Gap sign onto River Falls Road. Follow River Falls Road for about 6 miles as it winds around and changes to Jones Gap Road. From the parking lot, follow the short trail to the visitor center.

Lake Conestee Nature Preserve

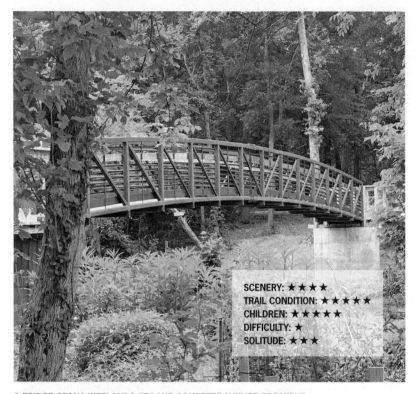

A BRIDGE SPANS WETLANDS AT LAKE CONESTEE NATURE PRESERVE.

SCENERY: ★★★★
TRAIL CONDITION: ★★★★★
CHILDREN: ★★★★★
DIFFICULTY: ★
SOLITUDE: ★★★

TRAILHEAD GPS COORDINATES: N34° 46.774' W82° 21.205'

DISTANCE & CONFIGURATION: 2.4-mile loop

HIKING TIME: 1.5 hours

HIGHLIGHTS: This is a designated wildlife sanctuary and regionally recognized birding hotspot with wetlands.

ELEVATION: 850' at trailhead, with no significant rise

ACCESS: Daily, sunrise–sunset; free, but $3 suggested donation

MAPS: Lake Conestee Nature Preserve, USGS *Mauldin*

FACILITIES: Restrooms (at baseball field), benches

WHEELCHAIR ACCESS: The preserve has 2 miles of paved trails accessible via wheelchair.

COMMENTS: Leashed dogs are allowed except on the east and west bay observations decks. Bikes are permitted on paved trails.

CONTACT: Lake Conestee Nature Preserve, 864-277-2004, conesteepreserve.org

Overview

Head here for an easy outdoor stretch on a Sunday afternoon or for an after-work escape. Located on the outskirts of Greenville, the preserve will make you feel as if you've just stepped into a jungle. With 6 miles of natural surface trails and 6 miles of paved trails, there is plenty to explore. The preserve is popular, so expect to meet up with others along the well-maintained route. After crossing the pedestrian bridge over the Reedy River, multiple paths and boardwalks traverse the wetlands. Birding aficionados will appreciate the observation decks, and wildlife is plentiful within the preserve.

Route Details

With Little League baseball fields lining the entrance to this 406-acre wildlife sanctuary, Lake Conestee Nature Preserve has become a popular place, especially on weekends. But don't let that deter you. There is plenty of room to seek solitude and enjoy nature.

Not only is the area scenic, it also has quite a bit of history. In the 1700s it was believed that the Cherokee used the Conestee area as a campsite while traveling. A mill was established in 1790, and then later became home to the Carruth Armory, the Patterson Paper Mill, and the McBee Manufacturing/ Reedy River Factory complex. By 1931 the mill and surrounding area had fallen into disrepair. There were prolonged legal issues surrounding pollution in the Reedy River, and the Great Depression took its toll on the area. Today the park is owned by the Conestee Foundation, a nonprofit organization committed to keeping Lake Conestee a nature preserve and wildlife sanctuary.

To begin this hike, start at the main entrance, E2 (Reedy River Bridge entrance), near the parking lot. Head west and cross the 215-foot expansion bridge over the Reedy River. This bridge was constructed in 2009 and provides an excellent view of the river and the surrounding forest.

Follow signs for the yellow trail, which heads south. In 2022, the preserve changed trail names, and while some of the former signs may remain, the paths are clearly marked with colored blazes. Several boardwalks sit atop wetlands, along with informational signs on the flora and fauna found in the preserve. This is the best place to spot urban wildlife such as deer, squirrels, birds, and rabbits.

Turn right (south) onto the connector, where a short walk takes you to the West Bay observation deck overlooking wetlands. From here you might see

Lake Conestee Nature Preserve

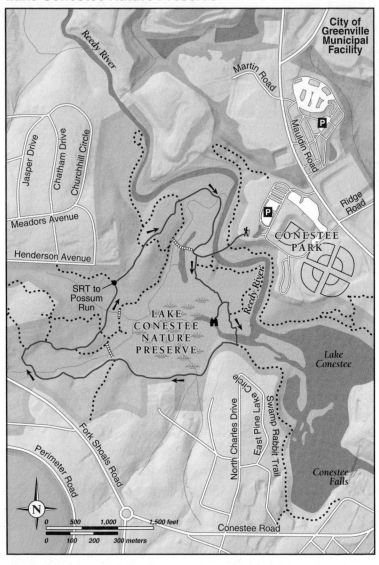

beaver dams, rusty blackbirds, raptors, piscivores, blue herons, ducks, geese, and cranes. More than 170 different bird species have been inventoried here by the Greenville County Bird Club and Audubon South Carolina. BirdLife International has designated Lake Conestee Nature Preserve as an Important Bird Area of Global Significance.

After leaving the observation deck, return to the yellow route and turn right, continuing south as you loop through the heavily forested land. Soon the green loop joins with the yellow trail, just before you cross a bridge. Turn right (west) to continue on the yellow trail as you join up with the north Swamp Rabbit Trail (SRT). As part of the southern extension of Greenville County's famed Prisma Health Swamp Rabbit Trail, the multiuse pathway is wide and paved here.

Continue along the SRT and yellow route, crossing several smaller connector trails as you wind through the preserve. When you get to a larger fork in the trail, continue toward the right (east), staying on SRT North and the yellow trail. You'll pass several additional trails, some color coded, but be sure to stay on the yellow route. When you reach the bridge over the Reedy River again, you will have completed a 2.4-mile loop.

Nearby Attractions

The trailhead is located at the home of **Greenville Little League Baseball.** You can access other trails that are part of the Lake Conestee Nature Preserve that will take you to **Conestee Village** and past the **Conestee Dam.** Parts of the trail combine with the **Prisma Health Swamp Rabbit Trail** system.

Directions

The main trailhead is at 840 Mauldin Road, Greenville. From I-85 take Exit 46/Mauldin Road and go south for about 2 miles. The park entrance will be on your right at the intersection of Braves Avenue and Mauldin Road. Drive past the baseball fields and turn right directly after the stadium. There is plenty of paved parking.

19

Paris Mountain State Park: Brissy Ridge Trail

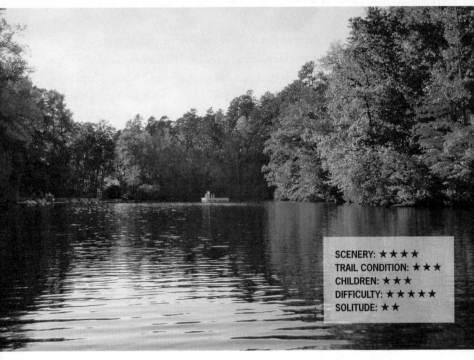

SCENERY: ★ ★ ★ ★
TRAIL CONDITION: ★ ★ ★
CHILDREN: ★ ★ ★
DIFFICULTY: ★ ★ ★ ★ ★
SOLITUDE: ★ ★

LAKE PLACID AT PARIS MOUNTAIN STATE PARK OFFERS FABULOUS FALL FOLIAGE.

TRAILHEAD GPS COORDINATES: N34° 56.452' W82° 23.277'

DISTANCE & CONFIGURATION: 3.1-mile loop

HIKING TIME: 2.5 hours

HIGHLIGHTS: Distant mountains, high elevation

ELEVATION: 1,495' at trailhead to 1,521' at top of ridge

ACCESS: Daily, 8 a.m.–8 p.m.; $6 for age 16 and older; $3.75 for SC seniors; $3.50 for children ages 6–15; free for age 5 and younger

MAPS: Paris Mountain State Park, USGS *Paris Mountain State Park*

FACILITIES: None at the trailhead; restrooms and picnic tables available in the park

WHEELCHAIR ACCESS: None

COMMENTS: Dogs are allowed but must be on a 6-foot leash at all times. During nice weather on weekends the area gets busy and parking might be a little hard to find. Mountain bikers and hikers share a portion of this trail except on Saturdays, when no mountain bikes are allowed on trails.

CONTACT: Paris Mountain State Park, 864-244-5565, southcarolinaparks.com/paris-mountain

Overview

Paris Mountain is easily one of Greenville's greatest assets. The close proximity to downtown Greenville makes this 1,540-acre park a nice family getaway, a place for a Sunday afternoon picnic, or even, in the summer, as an after-work retreat. The park features more than 15 miles of hiking/biking trails along with camping, fishing, and boating. With steep hills and twisting corners, the Brissy Ridge Trail offers a challenging hike with great mountain views, especially in the winter months, and is easily accessible.

Route Details

Paris Mountain is one of 16 state parks that were built by the Civilian Conservation Corps in South Carolina during the Great Depression. The visitor center is located in the renovated bathhouse and has historical exhibits, as well as classrooms where rangers teach children about the ecology and history of the park. Two of the four lakes at Paris Mountain were once used to supply water to Greenville.

The park is a monadnock, which is a mountain that rises up out of otherwise flat land, and has become a Greenville landmark. Paris Mountain is also very popular with bicyclists, who have full use of most of the trails and roadways except on Saturdays. George Hincapie and Lance Armstrong have both used Paris Mountain to train for the Tour de France.

To get to the trailhead, drive all the way to the top of Paris Mountain. There are two parking areas near the top. I prefer the topmost one, as there are more parking spaces available. From the trailhead in this lot, just follow the signs that say Brissy Ridge Trail. You will actually take a connector trail about half a mile to the trail. The connector trail follows alongside the road and heads right, slightly downhill. A small fork to the left leads to the road, so continue on the connector to the right.

When you get near the second parking lot, this is where the actual Brissy Ridge Trail begins. It's a loop trail, so either way is fine. We took the trail to the right, which turned out to be a good choice, as it meant tackling the steeper portions at the beginning of the hike instead of the end.

The route is well marked with signs and yellow trail markers on the trees. As you twist and turn down the mountain watch out for the many tree roots on the dirt trail. Be careful here—it only takes one root to make you lose your footing and take a tumble.

Paris Mountain State Park: Brlssy Ridge Trail

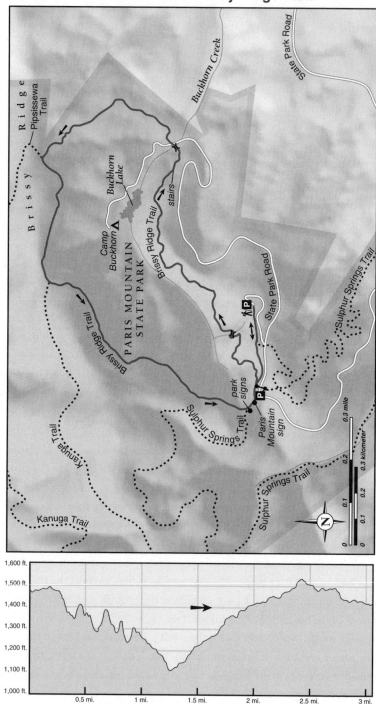

The trail continues mostly downhill with several switchbacks until you begin an even steeper descent. The path becomes much narrower here as you make your way alongside the mountain. As you cross a log that acts as a make-shift bridge over a small stream, look up at the trees that mark the hillside and see how far down you have come.

As you continue, the trail proceeds uphill for a short section before continuing downhill. There is a small stream to your left, and you can hear the faint sound of the water trickling its way down. Another uphill climb brings you around and back to the top of the mountain where you can glimpse the valley below through the trees.

As you round the corner, you immediately begin to descend again. The trail continues for a while with steep uphills followed by steep downhills. The path levels out for a short distance when you are once again at the top of the mountain ridge. As busy as this trail is, there are still periods of solitude.

The trees begin to thin out as you hear the rushing water and catch glimpses of the lake below. This is as close to the lake as you will get on this trail. A small wooden staircase helps lead you down the very steep descent here. Once at the bottom, you will cross a small bridge over a creek. On the other side after a short walk, you'll come to the park road.

Cross over the road, continuing to follow the yellow trail markers. Bikes are allowed on this portion of the trail, so it is wider and more level here. You will walk slightly uphill, crossing under some telephone poles until the trail begins to curve around and head back south.

As you continue mostly uphill, you will come to the top of the mountain ridge again. At 1.8 miles the Pipsissewa Trail comes in on the right, but you should continue west on the Brissy Ridge Trail. As you make your way alongside the mountain you will once again catch glimpses of the lake below. When you get to the top of the ridge again, enjoy the great peek-a-boo views through the trees of the city below and the mountains in the distance. Follow the path until you come to a fork in the trail.

At the fork, a sign indicates the Kanuga Trail to the right and the Brissy Ridge Trail to the left. Continue to the left, still following the yellow trail markers. In winter you can see for miles as you travel along the ridge of the mountain. The path is mostly even with only mild uphill and downhill sections, and soon you will come to the Brissy Ridge and Sulphur Springs trailhead and parking area. Unless you parked here, continue on the trail alongside this parking lot as you make your way to the upper parking lot and complete the loop.

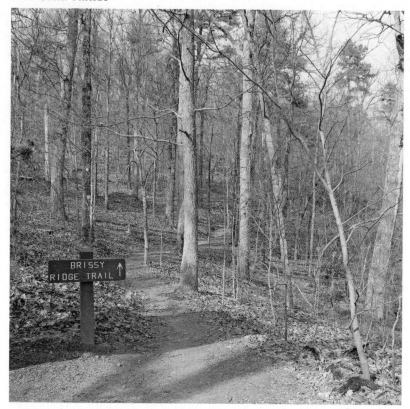

THE BRISSY RIDGE TRAIL IS WELL SIGNED.

Nearby Attractions

Paris Mountain State Park has four lakes and offers fishing at either the 8-acre **Lake Placid** or the 15-acre **Reservoir #3,** located at the back side of the park (you must hike in 2 miles to get to this lake). Canoes, kayaks, and pedal boats are available for rental depending on the weather and lifeguard availability at Lake Placid. There are eight other trails besides the Brissy Ridge Trail to hike, along with numerous places to picnic.

Directions

From I-385 take Exit 40 and turn left (north) onto Pleasantburg Road (SC 291). Go approximately 4 miles and then turn right onto Piney Mountain Road. Go to the first traffic light and turn right. The park entrance will be about 2 miles on the left.

20

Swamp Rabbit Trail: Cleveland Park to Linky Stone Park

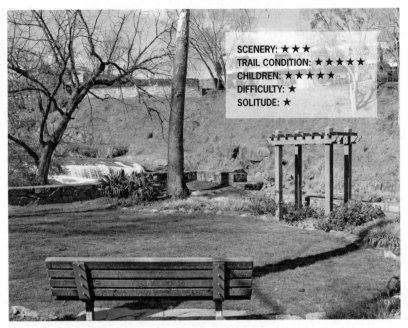

SCENERY: ★ ★ ★
TRAIL CONDITION: ★ ★ ★ ★ ★
CHILDREN: ★ ★ ★ ★ ★
DIFFICULTY: ★
SOLITUDE: ★

FALLS PARK IS A POPULAR DESTINATION FOR BOTH LOCALS AND VISITORS.

TRAILHEAD GPS COORDINATES: N34° 50.751' W82° 23.252'

DISTANCE & CONFIGURATION: 4.2-mile out-and-back, with a small balloon at end

HIKING TIME: 2.25 hours

HIGHLIGHTS: Downtown views, Falls Park, and the Reedy River Waterfall

ELEVATION: 827' at trailhead to 988' at Falls Park

ACCESS: Daily, sunrise–sunset; free

MAPS: Greenville Recreation, City of Greenville

FACILITIES: Public restrooms are located in Cleveland Park near the playground, at Falls Park near the waterfall, and at the Art Crossing area.

WHEELCHAIR ACCESS: Yes

COMMENTS: Dogs are welcome. Pet waste bags are located along the trail, as are water fountains for humans and dogs.

CONTACTS: Greenville Parks and Recreation Department, 864-288-6470, greenvillerec.com/swamprabbit; City of Greenville, 864-232-2273, greenvillesc.gov/316/Swamp-Rabbit-Trail

Swamp Rabbit Trail: Cleveland Park to Linky Stone Park

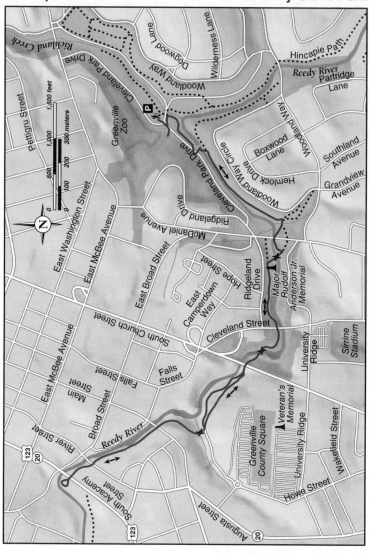

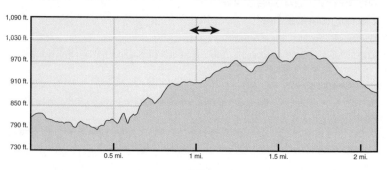

Overview

This urban oasis is downtown Greenville's crowning jewel. Bicyclists, hikers, families, and joggers all enjoy the 22-plus-mile multiuse trail system that turned an abandoned rail line into a greenway. The Prisma Health Swamp Rabbit Trail traverses Cleveland Park, a 126-acre urban park; Falls Park, a 40-acre downtown park situated on the site of an old sawmill in the heart of downtown Greenville's West End District; and Greenville's newest park, the 60-acre Unity Park. The Swamp Rabbit Trail connects nearby Travelers Rest with downtown Greenville and offers views of the Reedy River and Reedy River Falls.

Route Details

This route begins at the parking area just south of the playground at Cleveland Park and at the south end of the Greenville Zoo. There is no official trailhead here, but begin by following the Swamp Rabbit Trail signage, walking toward the Vietnam Veterans Memorial. You can walk many different paths, but this trail will take you through the nicest parts of Cleveland Park, alongside the Reedy River, into Falls Park with views of the waterfall, and down to Linky Stone Park and the Children's Garden.

As you walk along, you'll notice that joggers, bicyclists, and hikers all share the wide paved pathway. On nice days and weekends, the trail can be quite busy, but that is part of the fun. Greenville is a warm, welcoming town and people will often stop and say hello, allow furry friends to greet one another, and let children zoom on past.

When you come to a one-way double-pedestrian bridge, cross the Reedy River and follow along to the right on the paved pathway, continuing to follow the Swamp Rabbit Trail signs. Continue past several benches and a picnic shelter as you follow alongside the Reedy River to your right. At Picnic Shelter 3 you'll come to a fork. Take the small bridge to your right, following under McDaniel Avenue.

Veer to the right and take the Major Rudolf Anderson Jr. pedestrian bridge back over the river and past the Major Rudolf Anderson Jr. Memorial and U.S. Air Force plane. You'll cross under Cleveland Street as you continue following along with the river to your left now. When you come to another pedestrian bridge that crosses the river, cross over. Just on the other side of the bridge, you will pass under South Church Street and soon come to another fork in the trail at approximately 1.2 miles. Take the path to the right (northwest), following alongside with the Reedy River to your right. *Note:* This part of the trail is not ADA- or bike-friendly, so if you have a wheelchair, take the path to the left and it will eventually rejoin this trail.

You'll pass another picnic shelter, River Lodge Shelter #4, and benches will dot the pathway at frequent intervals at this point in the trail. A nice plaque and overlook commemorate Vardry Mill, the former textile mill that occupied this area in the late 1800s. The path splits here and you can go either way and end up in the same spot. To the left is a set of stone stairs and to the right is a smooth walkway.

Another set of stairs takes you up to the road, and this is where you will rejoin your wheelchair and bike friends. Right here is the best view of Reedy River Falls and the award-winning pedestrian suspension bridge that spans the falls. Turn right and cross the stone pedestrian bridge into the heart of Falls Park and the downtown West End District. It's quite busy here, with people enjoying picnics on the grassy lawn, dipping their toes into the Reedy River, and gazing at the magnificent waterfall.

THE SWAMP RABBIT TRAIL FOLLOWS THE REEDY RIVER IN SPOTS.

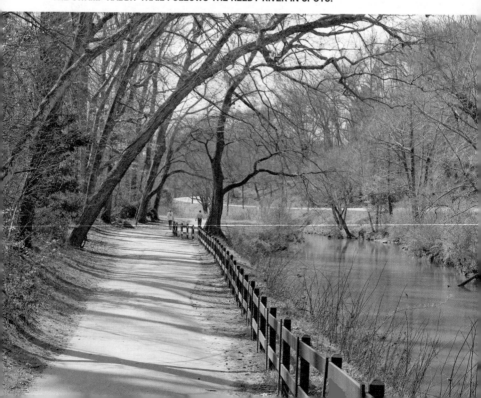

Continue on the pathway to the right, still following the Swamp Rabbit Trail signs. The trail continues with the Reedy River to the right as you come to the top of the falls. The route then passes under Main Street. The Art Crossing area will now be on your left; several artists have working/living spaces here. The trail continues as you cross over River Street. Be careful crossing here, as the road can be quite busy.

Just past River Street and right below Academy Street are Linky Stone Park and the Children's Garden at 1.9 miles into the trek. Check out the purple benches and picnic tables and references to popular children's books. Alphabet letters explain the different plant life, and the multithemed garden was designed to enrich children's creativity through exploration and discovery.

You could continue on the Swamp Rabbit Trail all the way to Travelers Rest, but that would be an additional 14 miles, so for this hike this is a good turnaround spot. To mix things up a little so the scenery isn't completely the same on the way back, take the trail back until you get to the pedestrian bridge in Falls Park. Then, continue straight instead of crossing the bridge up the left as you came. This is the alternate Swamp Rabbit Trail.

As you walk along this section, you'll notice a July 29, 2004, flood-level sign here indicating just how high the water from the Reedy River rose during a massive flooding. Follow the Swamp Rabbit Trail signs as the trail curves to the south, follows along Woodland Way, and then turns left after crossing the Reedy River. There are water fountains along this part of the path, but be aware that they are turned off in the winter. Once you get back to the trailhead parking lot you've completed the hike.

Nearby Attractions

Downtown Greenville offers restaurants, shopping, and minor league baseball. Bicycle rentals are available from several downtown vendors. **Cleveland Park** is home to the **Greenville Zoo** and offers picnic shelters, tennis and volleyball courts, playground areas, softball fields, and a fitness trail.

Directions

From downtown Greenville take Washington Street south for about 1 mile to Cleveland Park, 150 Cleveland Park Drive. Park in the parking lot just south of the playground, south of the zoo.

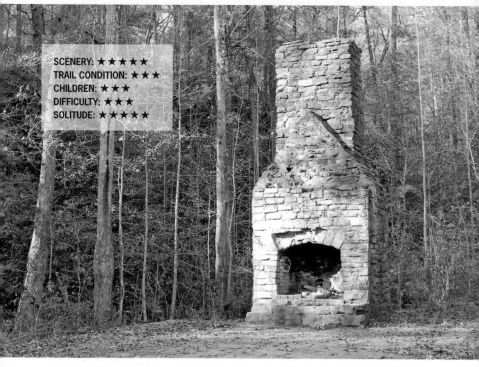

REMAINS OF A CCC STRUCTURE BUILT BETWEEN 1933 AND 1942

SCENERY: ★ ★ ★ ★ ★
TRAIL CONDITION: ★ ★ ★
CHILDREN: ★ ★ ★
DIFFICULTY: ★ ★ ★
SOLITUDE: ★ ★ ★ ★ ★

TRAILHEAD GPS COORDINATES: N35° 04.434' W82° 35.825'

DISTANCE & CONFIGURATION: 1-mile balloon

HIKING TIME: 1 hour

HIGHLIGHTS: Historic remains of building, three waterfalls

ELEVATION: 1,090' at trailhead to 1,204' about 0.25 mile into the hike at the top of the ridge

ACCESS: 24-7; free

MAPS: None

FACILITIES: None

WHEELCHAIR ACCESS: None

COMMENTS: Parking can be tight since it's just a pullout. There is no signage for the waterfall or the trail (OK, there is one small wooden sign on a tree). Locals also refer to this parking area as Wildcat Wayside. Due to a high number of accidents, the trail was reconstructed and takes a completely different path to the upper falls.

CONTACTS: 8155 Geer Highway (SC 11), Cleveland, SC 29635; The Learning Center for the Mountain Bridge Wilderness Area, 864-836-3647

Overview

A popular local spot for those heading to Table Rock State Park or Caesars Head State Park, the waterfalls here are the main draw. There are three waterfalls, with the first two accessible to just about everyone from the roadside. Visitors may not even realize they can take the moderate 1-mile loop trail and see the remains of a house and another taller waterfall. During the warmer months, on weekends, you can find the falls by looking for the hot-boiled-peanut vendor.

Route Details

It's one of the smaller waterfalls in South Carolina, but what Wildcat Branch Falls lacks in size (it's only about 30 feet high), it makes up for in fury. The waterfalls are fed by Wildcat Branch Creek, one of the South Saluda River tributaries. Once visitors step out of their car and approach the first of the falls, the sound of the highway evaporates and all that can be heard is the rush of the water falling over the rocks. Kick off your shoes and wade into the water. It's a welcome respite on a hot summer day.

There's more to see here than the initial waterfall, though, and this short, moderate trail is easy enough to traverse and leads to two more waterfalls as it travels through a secluded forest. The trail begins by following the set of stone stairs leading upward. Once up the stairs, you will see a second waterfall (the middle falls) to your left. This waterfall isn't as spectacular as the other two. It's only 10 feet tall, but the sound of the rushing water is soothing. Follow the stepping stones that take you across the small stream. The trail then leads to another stone staircase leading upward. Take the stairs, and the dirt path will level out as you walk a short way to the remains of a building. This structure was built by the Civilian Conservation Corps (CCC) sometime between 1933 and 1942. There are conflicting accounts of what the structure used to be. Some say it was a general building used by the CCC, while others say it was a home, and still others say it was a picnic structure. Whatever it was used for, all that remains today is the rock floor and chimney.

Continue making your way along the dirt trail and soon you will come to a fork. To the left is a wooden bridge across another small stream and to the right is a log and dirt staircase. This is where the loop portion of the trail begins. Take the staircase up and to the right. The pathway continues alongside the stream and along a ravine. The trees are thick here, with light barely filtering through.

Wildcat Branch Falls Trail

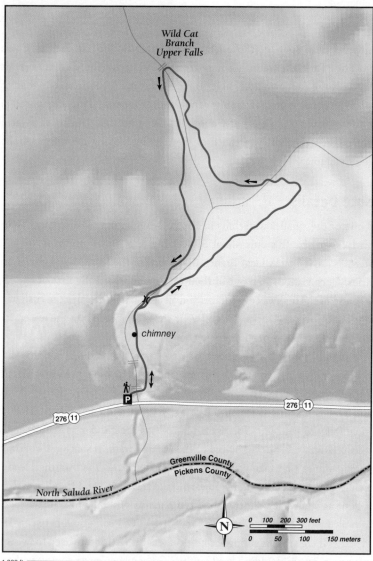

Wild Cat
Branch
Upper Falls

chimney

276 11

276 11

Greenville County
Pickens County

North Saluda River

0   100   200   300 feet
0   50   100   150 meters

N

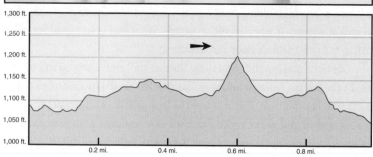

Make your way uphill as the stream below fades from sight. As you near the top of the hill, you'll also lose the sound of the rushing water, now far below.

Round a corner and then descend until you once again pick up the stream. Cross the stream using the well-positioned stepping stones and follow the trail deeper into the forest. At 0.6 mile you'll come upon the 100-foot upper waterfall. Depending on recent rainfall, it could be a magnificent cascade over the huge, flat granite boulder or just a thin line trickling down. As you leave the waterfall, the trail crosses the stream once again as it begins the loop back. Here you maneuver some boulders as you make your way downhill. Continue to follow the stream until you veer away to the right.

This area of the forest is very tranquil, with only the wind rustling the oak, hemlock, and pine trees and the smell of pine in the air. As you continue, you will follow a 10-foot cliff with the stream below. Descend for a short time until you come upon the wooden bridge, completing the loop portion of the trail. Backtrack past the CCC structure's remains as you complete your hike.

Nearby Attractions

Wildcat Branch Falls is close to **Table Rock State Park** and **Caesars Head State Park,** both of which have hiking trails, scenic views, and picnic areas.

Directions

From Greenville, go north on US 276. The trail is on the right side about 5 miles on SC 11 past the US 276/SC 11 junction. There is no signage, but there is a pullout and a small parking area.

Spartanburg and Cherokee Counties (Hikes 22–27)

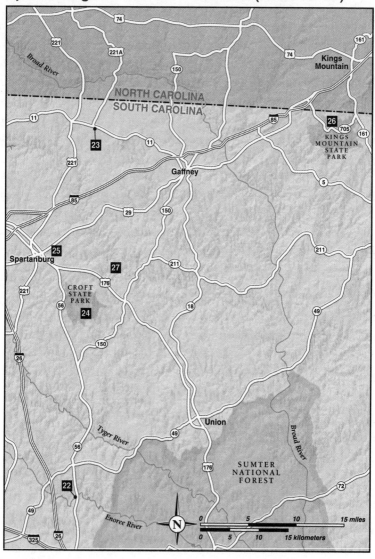

Spartanburg and Cherokee Counties

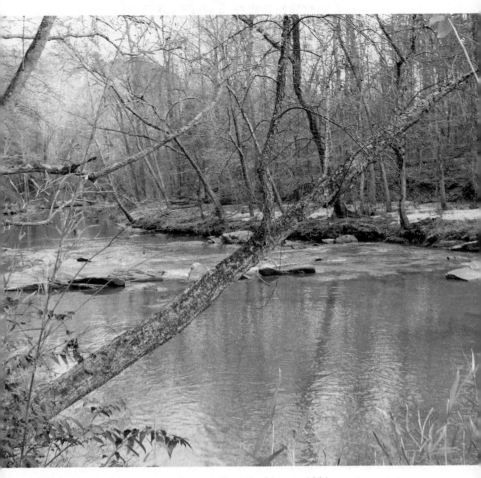

FAIRFOREST CREEK AT CROFT STATE PARK *(See Hike 24, page 126.)*

Battle of Musgrove Mill State Historic Site: British Camp and Battlefield Trails

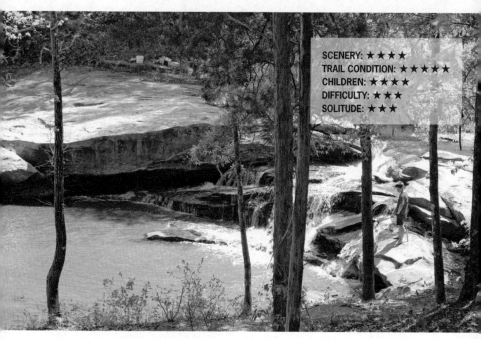

SCENERY: ★ ★ ★ ★
TRAIL CONDITION: ★ ★ ★ ★ ★
CHILDREN: ★ ★ ★ ★
DIFFICULTY: ★ ★ ★
SOLITUDE: ★ ★ ★

HORSESHOE FALLS AT MUSGROVE MILL

TRAILHEAD GPS COORDINATES:

> **Battlefield Trail** N34° 35.548' W81° 51.157'
> **British Camp Trail** N34° 35.811' W81° 51.321'

DISTANCE & CONFIGURATION: 2.3 miles, split between two trails; British Camp Trail is a loop, while Battlefield Trail is a balloon

HIKING TIME: Overall about 2 hours

HIGHLIGHTS: Interpretive trails depicting the 1780 British battle that took place here, great views of the Enoree River, and a small waterfall and swimming hole

ELEVATION: British Camp Trail, 396' at the lowest point and 524' at the highest; Battlefield Trail, 433' at the lowest point and 529' at the highest

ACCESS: Daily, 9 a.m.–6 p.m.; $3 for age 16 and older; $1.50 for SC seniors; $1 children ages 6–15; free for age 5 and younger

MAPS: Musgrove Mill State Historic Site, Musgrove Mill, USGS *Philson Crossroads*

FACILITIES: Restrooms and water fountain at the visitor center

WHEELCHAIR ACCESS: Accessible parking and 0.1-mile ADA-accessible trail to the waterfall at the Battlefield Trail only

COMMENTS: Dogs are allowed but must be on a 6-foot leash at all times. This is actually two different trails, and you will need to drive in between.

CONTACT: Musgrove Mill State Historic Site, 864-938-0100, southcarolinaparks.com/musgrove-mill

Overview

These are two distinctively different trails, but you can easily do them on the same day. British Camp Trail is a 1-mile leisurely hike that winds along the Enoree River. It offers views of where the old Musgrove mill and homesite used to be (unfortunately they washed away in 1852). The Battlefield Trail at Horseshoe Falls is about 1.3 miles and is a little more challenging; it takes you along an ancient gully and features the Revolutionary War site of the Battle of Musgrove Mill.

Route Details

Begin with the British Camp Trail, which starts at the parking lot sign at the visitor center. This trail loops through what was once the property of Edward Musgrove and the site of a temporary British encampment in 1780. Follow the cedar-lined trail by the picnic area. The trail descends from the picnic area into a meadow. Unfortunately, the route here is pretty close to the nearby highway and you can hear some traffic noise. But soon the path turns left to follow the Enoree River, and all outside noise will be gone. As the Enoree starts to rush faster and faster on the right, you'll see the remains of the old mill that belonged to Edward Musgrove. Several historical waysides along the trail denote points of interest, including the ruins of the Musgrove house, the Mary Musgrove Monument, the location of the 18th-century ford across the Enoree River, and the grist mill site. Continue along the river for about 0.3 mile until you begin a gradual uphill climb. Meander along the path until you come upon some picnic tables and a popular fishing pond. This hike takes about 45 minutes. You'll have to hop in the car and drive to the next hiking area. (See "Directions" on page 121.)

The Battlefield Trail starts across the street from the parking lot. Just a short walk from the trailhead is a lookout area with benches at Horseshoe Falls. The pool at the base of the small waterfall is a popular swimming hole. The first 0.1 mile of the trail is ADA accessible and paved. The trail is paved only to the falls; it becomes a natural trail after that. This is where you pick up the Battlefield Trail, which has interpretive signage explaining the Revolutionary War

Battle of Musgrove Mill State Historic Site: British Camp and Battlefield Trails

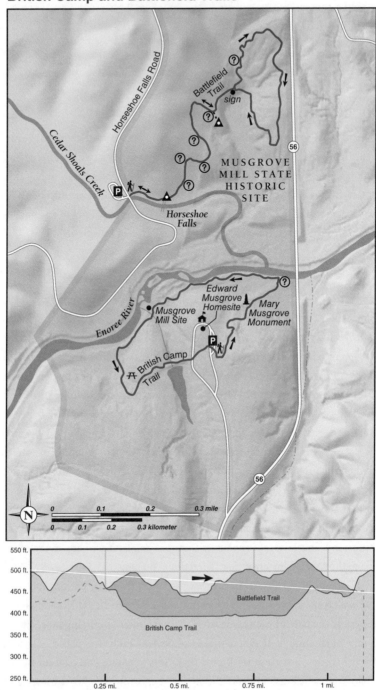

battle that took place here. Several historic waysides tell the story of the battle of the patriots and loyalists and the importance of the battle in the Revolutionary War. It's a very curvy trail but is well marked with green markings. The route is underused; even on a nice Saturday afternoon we were the only ones there. After the fifth interpretive sign you will come to a fork in the trail; head left. The trail follows an ancient gully where soldiers once hid and rose to battle. The trail winds around, and you'll follow close to the road for a little while. When cars aren't going by (it's not a busy road), it's easy to imagine you're back in the 1770s and the British are in hot pursuit. The trail ends at the Horseshoe Falls Road parking lot.

Nearby Attractions

The **Musgrove Mill Visitor Center** houses exhibits on the battle and some history of the American Revolution. It's a good place to stop in, pick up a map, and get familiar with the park.

Directions

The address is 398 State Park Road in Clinton. From I-26 take the Cross Anchor/ Clinton exit. Drive about 6 miles to the park entrance. To get to the Battlefield Trail turn left onto SC 56 from the visitor center. Drive about 1.5 miles until you get to Horseshoe Falls Road. Take a sharp left onto Horseshoe Falls Road and go another 1.5 miles. The parking lot will be on your right.

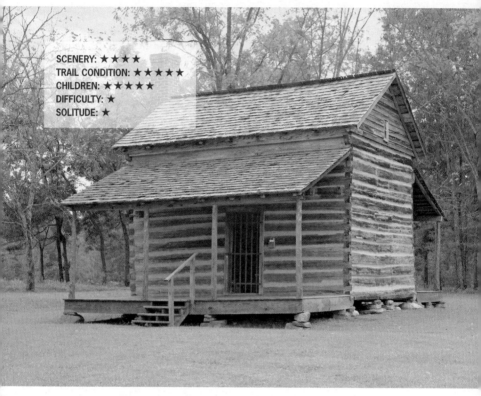

THE SCRUGGS HOUSE AT COWPENS NATIONAL BATTLEFIELD

SCENERY: ★ ★ ★ ★
TRAIL CONDITION: ★ ★ ★ ★ ★
CHILDREN: ★ ★ ★ ★ ★
DIFFICULTY: ★
SOLITUDE: ★

TRAILHEAD GPS COORDINATES: N35° 08.215' W81° 49.080'

DISTANCE & CONFIGURATION: 1.2-mile loop

HIKING TIME: 1 hour

HIGHLIGHTS: Easy trail with lots of history

ELEVATION: 1,059' at trailhead, with no significant elevation change

ACCESS: Daily, 9 a.m.–5 p.m.; trailhead parking lot: daily, sunrise–sunset; auto loop road and picnic area: daily, 9 a.m.–4:30 p.m.; free

MAPS: nps.gov/cowp

FACILITIES: Restrooms at the visitor center; picnic tables throughout the park

WHEELCHAIR ACCESS: Yes

COMMENTS: Dogs are allowed but must be leashed and are not allowed inside the visitor center. There is plenty of parking at the visitor center.

CONTACT: Cowpens National Park, 864-461-2828, nps.gov/cowp

Overview

This is really more of a walk than a hike, but the historical value makes it a definite inclusion for our five-star trails. Even though the Battle of Cowpens lasted less than an hour, it was the most significant turning point in the Revolutionary War, leading to the patriots' victory at Yorktown. On January 17, 1781, General Daniel Morgan led his outnumbered troops against British soldiers and won. Interpretive signs along the trail explain the important events that took place at this former cattle pasture (hence the name Cowpens). Bring the whole family on this historically significant trail.

Route Details

The trail begins behind the visitor center just to the left. Be sure to stop in and tour its museum, which has a reproduction of a three-pounder cannon along with other Revolutionary War weapons and exhibits. A huge fiber-optic display map illustrates the Southern Campaign of the American Revolution and the battle tactics employed by Captain Daniel Morgan at Cowpens. Morgan chose this land for its tactical advantage, with a river to the rear to discourage the ranks from breaking, rising ground on which to post his regulars, and an open forest and marsh on one side to thwart flanking maneuvers. A great 18-minute film, *Cowpens: A Battle Remembered,* depicts the battlefield events and is shown hourly.

Once you learn the history, head out the back door of the visitor center to the Cowpens Battlefield Trail. It begins as a paved pathway, but when you reach the historic Green River Road, it turns to dirt. Not only is this road where the British and Americans fought the Battle of Cowpens, it was also the main road that both sides took to get through the cowpens. It was used later as a gathering place for soldiers who fought the Battle of Kings Mountain. Prior to the Revolutionary War the road was used by settlers and Native Americans as a wagon and market trail.

The trail turns right and follows along the historic road. It begins a slight descent but levels out quickly and stays fairly level for the remainder of the route. Pasture fields dotted with trees expand on both sides of the path, and every 200 feet or so there are interpretive signs depicting the battlefield history. Some stops have metal statues of soldiers with wooden rifles that kids can use. Concrete footprints on the ground allow you to stand where the infantry would have stood to fire during the battle. Revolutionary War cannons dot the

Cowpens Battlefleld Trail

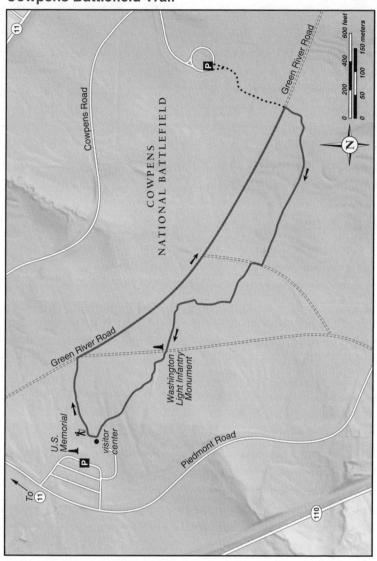

landscape to the right. At about the halfway point, when the trail begins to loop back, you'll come upon an intersection. Here you could continue walking along Green River Road, which leads to the Scruggs House (a preserved 1828 home that was moved to this site), but instead take a right and continue on the paved Battlefield Trail and visit the house later.

As you continue to walk through the quiet woodlands you may see deer, raccoons, squirrels, or other wildlife. Cowpens National Battlefield includes more than 842 acres of land and is home to a variety of plant and animal life. Its unique ecosystems and diverse habitats were crucial in the planning and success of the Battle of Cowpens. You'll also walk past the 1856 Washington Light Infantry Monument, the first monument placed on the Battle of Cowpens site in 1856. This steel monument with a concrete base and ball on the top isn't much to look at. Once past the monument you have only another quarter mile or so until you return to the visitor center.

The Battle of Cowpens was over in less than an hour but was a significant turning point in the Revolutionary War. After the battle was over and the wounded were cared for and the dead were buried, General Morgan knew that Cornwallis would come after them, so he led his troops northwest to camp alongside the Broad River. The next morning, he and his army resumed their journey, eventually stopping at Gilbert Town and continuing on to Kings Mountain.

For a longer hike you could consider walking the 3.8-mile auto-loop trail or the 2-mile Nature Trail. Every January, the park celebrates the anniversary of the battle with firing demonstrations and a living history encampment.

Nearby Attractions

The 3.8-mile one-way auto loop is a great way to view the perimeter of the battlefields and see the Scruggs House.

Directions

From Greenville or Spartanburg, take I-85 North to Exit 83. Turn left onto SC 110 and drive about 8 miles. Turn right onto SC 11 and the park will be on your right in about 0.5 mile.

24

Croft State Park Nature Trail

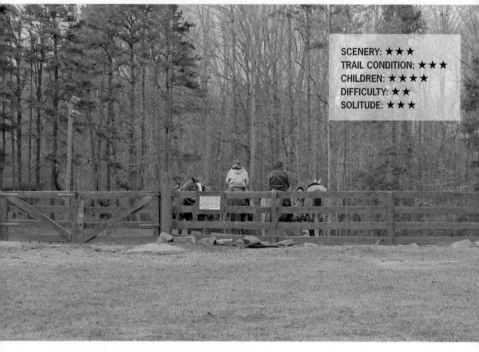

SCENERY: ★ ★ ★
TRAIL CONDITION: ★ ★ ★
CHILDREN: ★ ★ ★ ★
DIFFICULTY: ★ ★
SOLITUDE: ★ ★ ★

EQUESTRIAN CENTER AT CROFT STATE PARK

TRAILHEAD GPS COORDINATES: N34° 51.711' W81° 50.289'

DISTANCE & CONFIGURATION: 1.9-mile balloon

HIKING TIME: 1.25 hours

HIGHLIGHTS: Views of Fairforest Creek

ELEVATION: 604' at trailhead to 682' about 1.4 miles into the hike

ACCESS: Daily, 7 a.m.–6 p.m. Daylight saving time, daily, 7 a.m.–9 p.m.; $3 for age 16 and older; $1.50 for SC seniors; $1 for children ages 6–15; free for age 5 and younger

MAPS: Croft State Park

FACILITIES: Restrooms available near the first parking area. Horse stalls are available for rent.

WHEELCHAIR ACCESS: None

COMMENTS: Dogs are allowed but must be leashed. Bring insect repellent during warmer months.

CONTACT: Croft State Park, 864-585-1283, southcarolinaparks.com/croft

Overview

Located a few miles from downtown Spartanburg, Croft State Park is best known for its equestrian facilities, which boast an arena, on-site horse stalls, and more than 20 miles of equestrian trails. But this former Army training base also has more than 20 miles of hiking and biking trails, and the nature trail with interpretive signs is a great place to take the kids. Be sure to stay on the trails though and not to disturb unfamiliar objects on the off chance that the former infantry camp left something behind.

Route Details

Situated on the banks of Lake Tom Moore Craig, this park is a horse lover's paradise. Horse shows are held the third Saturday of each month (excluding December and January), so it's best to plan your hike accordingly, as the area can get busy during this time. The 7,054-acre park was an Army training base in the 1940s and once housed more than 250,000 soldiers. The training facility was closed in 1947 and reopened in 1949 as a state park.

The nature trail begins at the second trailhead, down the dirt road, past the equestrian arena, and past the no-day-use parking sign. While all of the trails here are open to hiking, this is one of the few trails in the park that does not share space with horses or bikes; it is foot-traffic only. As you begin down the dirt pathway, interpretive signs with photos and descriptions of the varied plant life appear every couple of feet. The trail is well marked and mostly quiet, with the exception of the sounds of the nearby shooting range cutting into the silence. Tall pine and hardwood trees are dense in some areas and sparser in others but still provide plenty of shade and canopy even in winter months.

As you continue along the mostly level trail, you will notice a river off to the right. This is Fairforest Creek. At the fork the trail begins its loop, and you can go either way; this description follows to the right. As you proceed, the river will be on your right as you approach the banks.

As you walk along the babbling creek, you'll see three wooden steps that lead downhill and even closer to the water's edge. The path becomes sandier here as you make a sharp left and head away from the river, slightly uphill.

The trail is still well marked with orange arrows as you continue uphill slightly. The interpretive signs have disappeared, but you can still hear the river and sometimes glimpse it through the trees. Soon cross over a small footbridge

Croft State Park Nature Trail

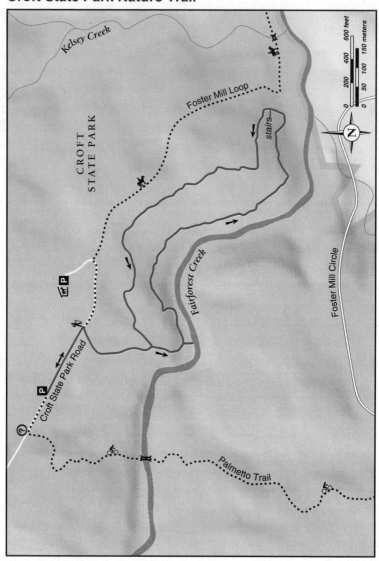

and then another until you are walking alongside the river again, this time a bit higher on the side of a hill instead of right next to it.

The trail gets pretty narrow here alongside the hill. Cross another small footbridge as you start to descend slightly. Cross yet another small bridge before you begin to go slightly uphill and then downhill again. The path curves to the left as you travel away from the river, and then becomes wider as it levels out.

You'll come to a rusting old iron bridge on the right. Continue on the path to the left until you reach some wooden stairs that lead back up the hill at approximately 1 mile. As you head back, you'll walk through the hardwood forest. The trail is level here and you can still hear the river faintly in the distance. Descend sharply again until you arrive back to where you began the loop portion of the trail. Turn right to head back toward the trailhead.

It's not uncommon to see deer, squirrels, snakes, and raccoons. Even foxes and coyotes have been spotted in the varying wildlife habitats.

This trail has some ups and downs, but the interpretive signs at the beginning and Fairforest Creek make it a great hike for kids.

Nearby Attractions

This park is located just a few miles from downtown Spartanburg and offers camping, equestrian trails, fishing, and boating. Near the entrance of the park is a small graveyard with historic gravesites.

Directions

From Spartanburg, take SC 56 to Dairy Ridge Road. Turn left, drive 0.3 mile, and then turn right onto Croft State Park Road. Drive through the park to the parking area just past the office, near the horse arena. There is another small parking area off the dirt road, just past the arena.

25

Edwin M. Griffin Nature Preserve

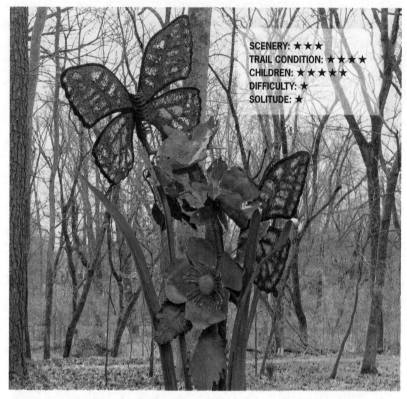

THIS SCULPTURE IS NEAR THE TRAILHEAD AT EDWIN M. GRIFFIN NATURE PRESERVE.

SCENERY: ★★★
TRAIL CONDITION: ★★★★
CHILDREN: ★★★★★
DIFFICULTY: ★
SOLITUDE: ★

TRAILHEAD GPS COORDINATES: N34° 57.170' W81° 53.508'

DISTANCE & CONFIGURATION: 4.2-mile bouquet-of-balloons configuration

HIKING TIME: 2.5 hours

HIGHLIGHTS: Urban trail, Lawson's Fork Creek, wetlands area

ELEVATION: 773' at trailhead, with no significant elevation change

ACCESS: Daily, sunrise–sunset; free

MAPS: spartanburgconservation.org

FACILITIES: Pet waste bags available; benches and picnic tables

WHEELCHAIR ACCESS: On portions of the trail

COMMENTS: Dogs allowed but must be leashed. Bring insect repellent in warmer months.

CONTACT: Spartanburg Area Conservancy, 864-948-0000, spartanburgconservation.org/cottonwood-trail

Overview

Edwin M. Griffin Nature Preserve was the Spartanburg Area Conservancy (SPACE) program's first project. This 115-acre urban preserve and trail system is located just minutes from downtown Spartanburg and follows Lawson's Fork Creek. The preserve serves as an important water quality buffer and offers a habitat for squirrels, deer, raccoons, and many other animals. Signage along the trails identifies some of the 50-plus tree species, and a 500-foot boardwalk and observation deck allow visitors to observe the wetlands area.

Route Details

This hike traverses pretty much every trail in the preserve. There are many different combinations and directions that you can go in the preserve, which makes it a great destination to hike as little or as much as you want. It's an easy walk and a great place to bring the kids and dogs on a Sunday afternoon or even after school or work during the week.

Start at the trailhead by the flower sculpture and take the mulched pathway to the right (southwest). You'll be following the Cottonwood Trail, and there are several benches and picnic tables in this area, making it a great place either before or after the hike to have a nice lunch or snack. There's also a small outdoor amphitheater area that was built as an Eagle Scout project. The pathways are very popular with joggers, so be sure to use proper trail etiquette.

Continue along the path until you come to a footbridge crossing Lawson's Fork Creek. Cross over the creek as the path turns to the right, heading underneath Fernwood Drive with the creek to your left. The roadway can be busy at times, and the traffic sounds are a reminder that you are still in the middle of the city. The path narrows and turns to dirt as you cross under the road. The river becomes wider, and houses dot the overlooking landscape. The sound of birds and the creek, though, begin to make it feel like the urban oasis it is. Approximately 0.5 mile into the trek, when you come to another bridge crossing over a smaller stream, take it.

Directly across the bridge, the trail forks into a balloon section of the trail. Here you head to the left (west), continuing alongside the quiet creek. As the distance between the nearby homes and the trail begins to widen, the hike becomes more serene.

Bird feeders dot the banks of the creek, providing a haven for birds. A bench and a staircase leading down to a small beach area mark where the trail

Edwin M. Griffin Nature Preserve

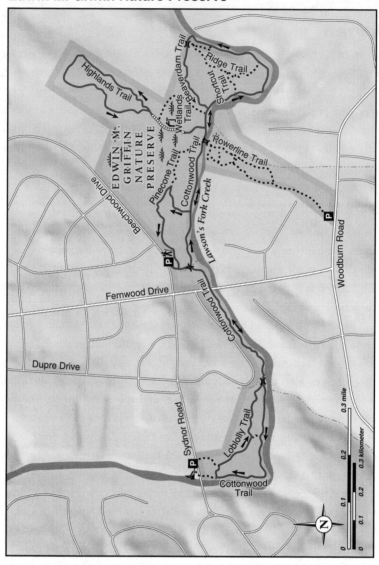

begins to curve right, toward the end of this balloon section. Continue with the creek to your left and you soon come to another fork. The outside trail leads under Sydnor Road, to another parking area for the preserve and to a kayak put-in spot that is part of the Lawson's Fork Paddling Trail. It's okay to head up there and explore, but be sure to come back to the fork and take the trail to the right (southeast).

When you come to another trailhead, a sign indicates that Cottonwood Trail is the way you just came, and Loblolly Trail is to the right. Follow the Loblolly Trail sign. While there are some trail signs, you'll notice that they are few and far between. You'll also notice signs on some of the trees, identifying some of the more than 50 species in the preserve. As you pass by tulip poplar, river birch, Carolina silver bell, and hackberry trees, you can appreciate just how many different trees are in this forest.

You'll soon complete this balloon portion as you meet back up with the Cottonwood Trail. Follow the Cottonwood Trail back until you get to the first bridge you crossed. Take the trail now to your right. This path turns away from the creek for just a short while but soon returns to the water.

This part of the trail feels more serene as nearby homes are a little more in the distance, shielded by trees. Several benches alongside the river allow you to sit and enjoy nature and the view. At another fork in the trail, you'll come to a nice footbridge that crosses the creek. On the other side of the creek is an open space with several picnic tables. This is a great place to have lunch and let the kiddos run wild. There is also a small disc-golf course here.

At the bridge the path forks again and either heads left with a sign that reads wetlands or continues straight ahead. Continue straight ahead, still following along the river, going under the power lines. You will be on the outer edge of the wetlands area. This area is wide and marshy and features an open clearing with a butterfly garden on the right.

There are several turnoffs, but continue to follow along the river on the outside edge of the preserve. You'll soon be under the canopy of the tall hardwood trees once again. When you get to a sign that reads Ridge Trail, ignore it, and continue on the path straight ahead. You'll come to a small bridge and then the path will immediately turn left (west), making this the next portion of a balloon. Here you'll turn away from the river as you begin to follow a small tributary.

The path becomes narrower with a hillside on your left and the stream to the right. But that doesn't last long, and soon the path widens again as you continue through the hardwood forest. You'll finish that loop and then head back by the butterfly garden. At the power line tower, veer to the right at the walkway sign. This is a shortcut that will meet up with the Wetlands Trail.

Take the Wetlands Trail to the right and cross the long footbridge atop the wetlands area. Signs placed along the bridge show some of the animals that inhabit this area, such as opossum and woodpeckers. At 3.1 miles, there is a nice observation platform in the middle of the long walkway with benches where you can sit and take in the surrounding area.

Before you get to the end of the bridge, a smaller footbridge goes to the right, but continue straight ahead (north). The trail proceeds slightly uphill to another fork. Continue on the trail straight and toward the right. More tree signs identify the sugar berry and red mulberry trees. As you cross over a dirt roadway, pine trees predominate, and pine needles litter the ground.

As the trail begins its next balloon, there is another access point off to the right, but you continue on the trail to the left to complete this loop. You never quite leave the sounds of civilization behind in this hike, but every so often you'll have a peaceful moment. Cross the dirt road again and follow signs for the Highlands Trail, which goes uphill again, making this the steepest portion of the hike.

After coming to a small overlook area, follow the path back the way you came until you get to another turnoff to the right. Follow this path to the right as it leads you back the way you came for a little bit and then veers left to follow the Pinecone Trail, which leads back to the parking area and concludes the hike.

Nearby Attractions

This trail is just minutes from downtown Spartanburg. **Croft State Park** and the **Pacolet Heritage Preserve** also offer hiking opportunities. Along the trail there is a kayak put-in; depending on creek conditions, kayaking might be an option.

Directions

From I-26 in Spartanburg, take US 29 East. Drive approximately 6 miles and then turn right onto Fernwood Drive. Drive about half a mile and then turn left onto Beechwood Drive. The gravel parking area will be on the right.

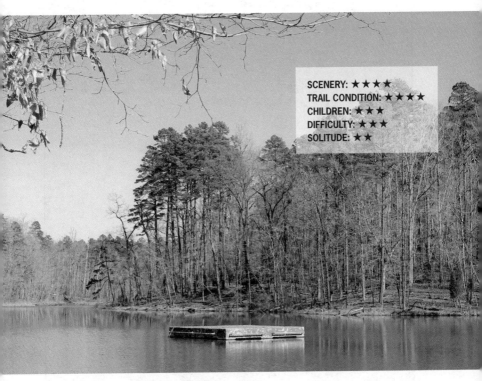

SCENERY: ★ ★ ★ ★
TRAIL CONDITION: ★ ★ ★ ★
CHILDREN: ★ ★ ★
DIFFICULTY: ★ ★ ★
SOLITUDE: ★ ★

LAKE CRAWFORD AT KINGS MOUNTAIN STATE PARK

TRAILHEAD GPS COORDINATES: N35° 08.484' W81° 22.559'

DISTANCE & CONFIGURATION: 6.6-mile out-and-back

HIKING TIME: 5 hours

HIGHLIGHTS: Historically significant battlefield site and views of Lake Crawford

ELEVATION: 864' at trailhead to 923' at 0.4 mile into the hike

ACCESS: Daily, 9 a.m.–5 p.m.; Memorial Day–Labor Day: Daily, 9 a.m.–6 p.m.; free

MAPS: Kings Mountain NPS, Kings Mountain State Park

FACILITIES: Restrooms, vending machine, and museum located at the visitor center. Picnic areas, camping, boat rentals, and equestrian facilities located throughout both parks.

WHEELCHAIR ACCESS: The 1.5-mile Battlefield Loop Trail is paved and has wheelchair access, but Kings Mountain National Recreation Trail does not.

COMMENTS: Dogs are allowed but must be leashed. Be sure to register at the visitor center before hiking any of the backcountry trails.

CONTACTS: Kings Mountain State Park, 803-222-3209, southcarolinaparks.com/kings-mountain; Kings Mountain National Military Park, 864-936-7921, nps.gov/kimo

Kings Mountain

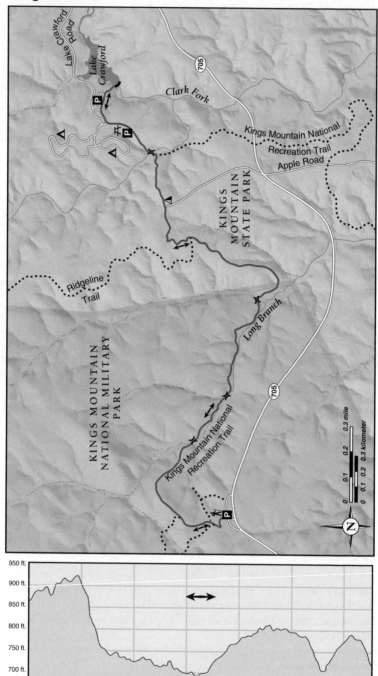

Overview

You get two parks in one at Kings Mountain: Kings Mountain National Military Park, which has a museum and visitor center and is home to the actual battlefield site; and the adjacent Kings Mountain State Park, which has two lakes, camping and equestrian facilities, and a living history farm. As the first major patriot victory, the Battle of Kings Mountain, which took place October 7, 1780, was considered a major turning point in the Revolutionary War. Thomas Jefferson called it "the turn of the tide of success," and while hiking in the park, it's easy to picture yourself as a Revolutionary soldier, getting ready for the battle.

Route Details

This hike goes through both Kings Mountain National Military Park and Kings Mountain State Park, but you won't even know when you're crossing from one to the other. In addition to the historical component, the parks offer amazing views and lush creeks and lakes. Most trails leave from the national park visitor center, and there is ample parking. Note that the parking area closes at 5 p.m., so plan accordingly.

Begin the hike on the paved Battlefield Loop Trail, directly to the right of the visitor center. When you get to the Victory Garden, turn right at the BACK COUNTRY TRAIL sign and follow the blue blazes of the Kings Mountain National Recreation Trail (NRT). The trail veers left (north) as a gravel access road goes to the right. Stay on the trail. There are several handmade wood benches here to sit on, but you shouldn't need a break so soon. The well-maintained path begins as a dirt and gravel path but turns to just dirt.

Kings Mountain NRT heads slightly uphill through the trees until you get to a fork. To the left will take you on the Browns Mountain Trail, a 2.4-mile out-and-back, but you should continue straight on the mostly level trail. You will notice you are now walking on top of the ridge of Kings Mountain with other ridgelines visible through the trees to the right and the left.

As you begin a slight descent, the trail becomes littered with tree roots and rocks, but it's still well marked and well maintained. As you go farther downhill, you begin to hear a babbling creek and the trees become more lush. The creek is called both Long Branch Creek and Clark's Creek, and even the park rangers on-site had no idea why it has two names. A nice wooden footbridge crosses the creek. Continue walking along the mostly level path with the stream to your right.

You will come across another wooden footbridge passing over a smaller stream. At 1 mile the trail is even closer to the creek, following directly alongside it. As you get deeper into the park it's easy to imagine you're a soldier camping on the banks of the river waiting for orders to attack. Even on busy days it's still very tranquil here. During spring, wildflowers dot the landscape, while winter months bring better views through the bare trees.

Another large, flat wooden bridge crosses the creek again as you continue on the mostly level path. As you leave the creek behind, you begin uphill for just a short distance until the path once again levels out. Quartz rocks are prominent along the path, and as you walk along there is a ravine to the right with the sound of tree frogs croaking in the background. Continue through the hardwood forest where the trees are sparse but plentiful.

At 2 miles you come to a bench and another sign. This is where the Ridgeline Trail branches off to the left (west). Continue forward on the Kings Mountain

A BRIDGE CROSSING AT KINGS MOUNTAIN

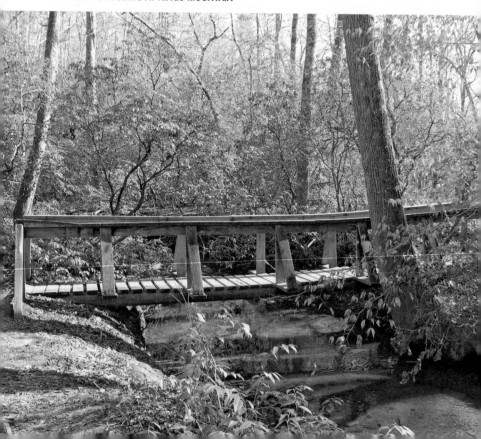

NRT and you'll soon come to a parking area for the remote/scout campsite. It's 0.3 mile to the lake from here. Continue following the blue trail signs toward Lake Crawford.

The path heads downhill and is moderately steep in a short section. At a fork you'll come to a wooden bridge to take you across the creek. If you were to go straight ahead, it would take you on the 16-mile loop trail. Continue to the left, over the bridge and then to the left again. The trail heads uphill, leaving the creek below.

At the top of the hill, there are picnic shelters, restrooms, and another parking area. Continue walking to the right along the road, cutting through the picnic area to a lower parking lot. Walk through the parking lot to the right, and just past the farm trail sign you'll come to the old bathhouse. Here there are great views of Lake Crawford and the dam that formed the lake. This is where you turn around and hike back the way you came. Overall, this trail is fairly easy with just a few slightly steep ups and downs, but this hike gets a moderate rating due to the length.

Nearby Attractions

Kings Mountain has several other hiking trails. The 1.5-mile paved **Battlefield Loop Trail** travels along where the Battle of Kings Mountain was fought and provides insight into both the patriot and loyalist camps during the famous skirmish. There's also a living-history farm, equestrian facilities, and two lakes that offer boating and swimming at the state park. A 16-mile park loop trail and the 1.8-mile **Ridgeline Trail** connect three parks and the states of North and South Carolina.

Directions

From I-85 take Exit 2 in North Carolina and go south on SC 216, reentering South Carolina. Follow the signs to the park.

Pacolet River Heritage Trust Preserve: Lawson's Fork Trail

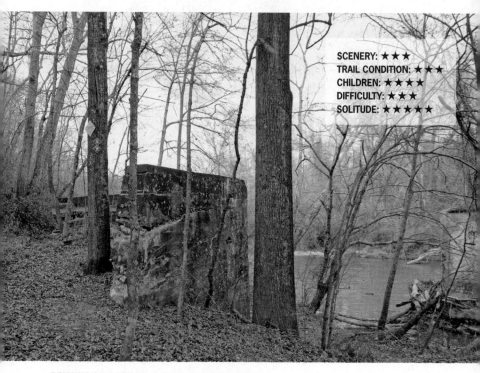

SCENERY: ★★★
TRAIL CONDITION: ★★★
CHILDREN: ★★★★
DIFFICULTY: ★★★
SOLITUDE: ★★★★★

REMAINS OF A BRIDGE ALONG THE PACOLET RIVER

TRAILHEAD GPS COORDINATES: N34° 55.786' W81° 46.858'

DISTANCE & CONFIGURATION: 2.9-mile balloon

HIKING TIME: 2 hours

HIGHLIGHTS: 3,500-year-old soapstone quarries and views of the Pacolet River

ELEVATION: 679' at trailhead to 720' at peak near the beginning of the trail

ACCESS: Daily, sunrise–sunset; free

MAPS: spartanburgconservation.org

FACILITIES: None

WHEELCHAIR ACCESS: None

COMMENTS: Dogs are allowed but must be leashed. Bring insect repellent in warmer months.

CONTACT: DNR Heritage Preserve Program, 803-734-3886, www2.dnr.sc.gov/ManagedLands

Overview

This 278-acre preserve was formed in 1993 by the Heritage Trust Program to protect the land as well as two prehistoric Native American soapstone quarries that provide a unique habitat for a variety of uncommon plants such as moss and leafy liverwort. The trail offers great views of the Pacolet River and is close enough to downtown Spartanburg to be enjoyed after work or on a nice Sunday afternoon. In the spring and fall, migrating songbirds use the preserve as a nesting spot.

Route Details

This 2.9-mile balloon trail combines two trails in this 278-acre preserve. A good portion of the trail snakes along the Pacolet River, and wildlife can often be seen along the way. The trailhead begins at the parking area where there are two trail signs, one that is small and green and reads HERITAGE TRUST and another white one that reads TRAIL. Begin the hike by following the green trail sign and proceed through the white gate.

The trail begins as a wide dirt pathway that is mostly level with hardwood trees on either side. When you get to a fork at 0.2 mile, turn left (north), following the green trail signs. As you follow the path, it becomes narrower but remains mostly level as the quietness envelops you. Only the birds can be heard chirping overhead. Hardwood trees still predominate, and don't be surprised if you see deer grazing in the distance.

The trail continues along the crest of a hill as it slopes downward on either side of you. Here you begin to descend slightly and to hear rushing water. The pathway becomes narrower and steeper as you continue downhill.

When you arrive at the bottom of the hill, there will be a bridge over a small stream and ravine. Cross the bridge as the trail continues to the right. The route goes slightly uphill and then downhill again as it winds around.

You can still hear rushing water, though it's no longer visible as the trail gets tougher and less even. Deer hoofprints dot the sandy parts of the trail, which is more of a water runoff than an actual path. But soon the trail levels out and you continue winding through the hardwood forest with lush vegetation and ferns all around.

When you come to the bank of the Pacolet River, the trail continues to the left. As you follow along the river, birds are more abundant. The river is calm, and there are several pathways that lead a little closer to the banks. As

Pacolet River Heritage Trust Preserve: Lawson's Fork Trail

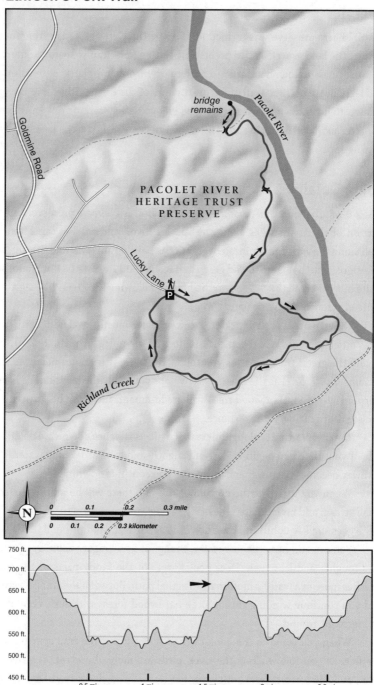

bridge
remains

Pacolet River

PACOLET RIVER
HERITAGE TRUST
PRESERVE

Goldmine Road

Lucky Lane

P

Richland Creek

| 0 | 0.1 | 0.2 | 0.3 mile |
| 0 | 0.1 | 0.2 | 0.3 kilometer |

N

750 ft.
700 ft.
650 ft.
600 ft.
550 ft.
500 ft.
450 ft.

0.5 mi.   1 mi.   1.5 mi.   2 mi.   2.5 mi.

you round the corner, the path turns to the left as you begin to head away from the river.

As you leave the river, you'll begin following a different small stream on your right. The trail goes steeply downhill again for a short distance until you come to a bridge and cross the same stream you were following.

Curve around for just a short distance until you get back to the river and see the remains of an old stone-and-concrete bridge at 0.9 mile into the hike. In 1903 torrential rains made the river rise 40 feet, washing the bridge away. The mill community here also lost more than 2,500 bales of cotton down the river, and 80 people died in the floodwaters.

This is the end of the trail, so turn around and go back the way you came until you get to the fork. Here, you take the trail marked with white trail signs to the left (east). The path is fairly level with a slight downhill, and soon you'll be walking along the top of two ravines, higher this time than at the beginning of the hike. As you reach the Pacolet River again, take a few minutes to enjoy the calm and serenity here. Soon the trail turns right and heads away from the river.

Next travel along a smaller tributary river, Richland Creek, on the left. There's a lot of bamboo here as the trail narrows but still follows alongside the river. Trail signs are not as prevalent, but you can still make out the path.

As you continue along the river, the trees are a little sparser. Soon the path turns left and immediately begins a fairly steep climb. When you reach the top of the ravine again, the parking lot comes into view and you conclude the hike.

Nearby Attractions

This trail is not too far from downtown Spartanburg. You can easily combine this hike with the **Croft State Park Nature Trail** (see page 126).

Directions

From Spartanburg, take US 176/SC 9 east for about 6.5 miles. Turn left onto Bethesda Road and cross Goldmine Road onto Nature View Lane. At the fork, turn right onto Lucky Lane. Drive to the end of the road and park in the parking area.

Appendix A:
Outdoor Retailers

APPALACHIAN OUTFITTERS
191 Halton Road
Greenville, SC 29607
864-987-0618
appoutfitters.com

CABELA'S
1025 Woodruff Road
Greenville, SC 29607
864-516-8100
cabelas.com

DICK'S SPORTING GOODS
1125 Woodruff Road
Greenville, SC 29607
864-284-6199
dickssportinggoods.com

THE LOCAL HIKER
173 E. Main St.
Spartanburg, SC 29306
864-764-1651
thelocalhiker.com

MAST GENERAL STORE
111 N. Main St.
Greenville, SC 29601
864-235-1883
mastgeneralstore.com

REI
1140 Woodruff Road, Ste. 400
Greenville, SC 29607
864-297-0588
rei.com

SOUTHERN APPALACHIAN OUTDOORS
319 Gentry Memorial Highway
Easley, SC 29640
864-507-2195
saopickens.com

SUNRIFT ADVENTURES
1 Center St.
Travelers Rest, SC 29690
864-834-5439
sunrift.com

Appendix B:
Hiking Clubs

The Upstate is home to several hiking clubs and groups that welcome you to contact them for specific hiking opportunities and other information.

GIRLS WHO HIKE SC
facebook.com/groups/GirlsWhoHikeSC

GREENVILLE NATURAL HISTORY ASSOCIATION HIKING CLUB
greenvillehiking.com

UPSTATE HIKING AND OUTDOOR ADVENTURES
meetup.com/upstate-hiking-and-outdoor-adventures

Y HIKING CLUB FOR YMCA OF EASLEY, PICKENS, AND POWDERSVILLE
pcymca.net

Y HIKING CLUB FOR YMCA OF GREATER SPARTANBURG
spartanburgymca.org/hiking-club

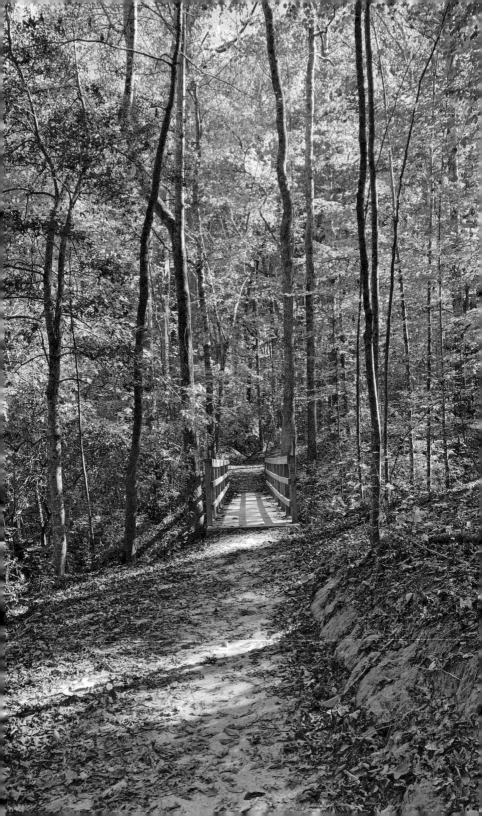

Index

Check out these great titles from
Adventure Publications!

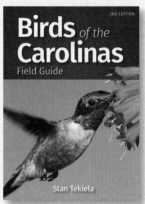

Birds of the Carolinas Field Guide

By Stan Tekiela
ISBN: 978-1-64755-068-4
$16.95, 3rd Edition
4.38 x 6, paperback
384 pages, color photographs

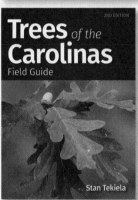

Trees of the Carolinas Field Guide

By Stan Tekiela
ISBN: 978-1-64755-071-4
$16.95, 2nd Edition
4.38 x 6, paperback
372 pages, color photographs

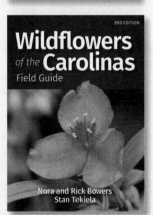

Wildflowers of the Carolinas Field Guide

By Nora and Rick Bowers and
    Stan Tekiela
ISBN: 978-1-64755-221-3
$18.95, 2nd Edition
4.38 x 6, paperback
432 pages, color photographs

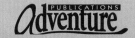

Check out this great title from
Menasha Ridge Press!

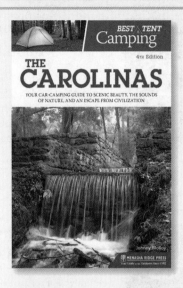

Best Tent Camping: The Carolinas

by Johnny Molloy
ISBN: 978-1-63404-151-5
$16.95, 4th Edition

6 x 9, paperback
Full color, 192 pages
Maps, photographs, index

The Carolinas provide spectacular backdrops for some of the most scenic campgrounds in the country. But do you know which campgrounds offer the most privacy? Which are the best for first-time campers? Johnny Molloy has traversed the entire region, from the alluring Blue Ridge Mountains to the saltwater-washed sands of the Atlantic coast, and compiled the most up-to-date research to steer you to the perfect spot! The full-color, updated, user-friendly format lets you easily find 50 of the best campgrounds to fit your travel plans and meet your personal interests, with author selections based on location, topography, size, and overall appeal.

Detailed maps of each campground and key information such as fees, restrictions, dates of operation, and facilities help to narrow down your choices, and ratings for beauty, privacy, spaciousness, safety and security, and cleanliness ensure that you find your perfect car-camping adventure. So whether you seek a quiet campground near a fish-filled stream or a family campground with all the amenities, *Best Tent Camping: The Carolinas* is a keeper.

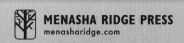

MENASHA RIDGE PRESS
menasharidge.com

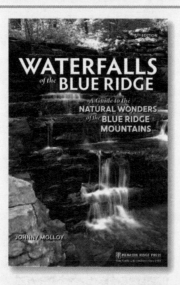
 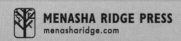

Check out this great title from
Wilderness Press!

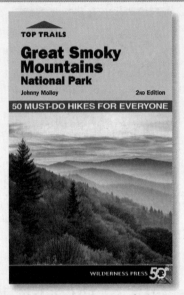

Top Trails: Great Smoky Mountains National Park

by Johnny Molloy   5 x 8
ISBN 13: 978-0-89997-876-5   416 pages, paperback
$18.95, 2nd Edition   photographs, maps, index

With its secluded mountain waterways, awe-inspiring views from grassy balds, diverse plant and animal life, and impressive stands of old-growth forest, Great Smoky Mountains National Park offers an overwhelming number of outdoor adventures. *Top Trails: Great Smoky Mountains National Park* describes both the park's classic destinations and lesser-known jewels in 50 must-do hikes. The trails range from an easy family stroll to a 7-mile trek through spruce forest atop a peaceful ridge to a panoramic 22-mile overnighter. Each entry in the book includes clear and concise directions, a detailed route map and elevation profile, "don't get lost" milestones, and expert trail commentary.

DEAR CUSTOMERS AND FRIENDS,

SUPPORTING YOUR INTEREST IN OUTDOOR ADVENTURE, travel, and an active lifestyle is central to our operations, from the authors we choose to the locations we detail to the way we design our books. Menasha Ridge Press was incorporated in 1982 by a group of veteran outdoorsmen and professional outfitters. For many years now, we've specialized in creating books that benefit the outdoors enthusiast.

Almost immediately, Menasha Ridge Press earned a reputation for revolutionizing outdoors- and travel-guidebook publishing. For such activities as canoeing, kayaking, hiking, backpacking, and mountain biking, we established new standards of quality that transformed the whole genre, resulting in outdoor-recreation guides of great sophistication and solid content. Menasha Ridge Press continues to be outdoor publishing's greatest innovator.

The folks at Menasha Ridge Press are as at home on a whitewater river or mountain trail as they are editing a manuscript. The books we build for you are the best they can be, because we're responding to your needs. Plus, we use and depend on them ourselves.

We look forward to seeing you on the river or the trail. If you'd like to contact us directly, visit us at menasharidge.com. We thank you for your interest in our books and the natural world around us all.

SAFE TRAVELS,

BOB SEHLINGER
PUBLISHER

About the Author

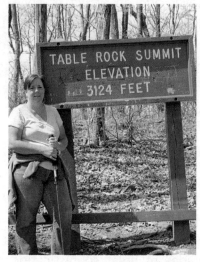

SHERRY JACKSON has a love of travel and exploration that began in childhood, when her family would load up the car on the weekend, pick a destination, and set off. Sherry has hiked through jungles, snorkeled the turquoise waters of the Caribbean, and wandered the streets of Paris, always searching for her next adventure. Growing up in Arizona, she joined her family on hikes into the Superstition Mountains and the Grand Canyon.

Sherry began writing for school newspapers and her own travel journals that portrayed her family's vacations. As an adult, she settled on a career in information technology—for a while. Today, she's vice president of content and digital for a local media company in Greenville, South Carolina. She has written hundreds of articles for national, regional, and local publications on topics such as business, travel, technology, and more.